# HIATAL HERNIA DIET FOR OVER 40

A Comprehensive Guide, Featuring Delicious Organic and Gluten-Free Options, Holistic Healing Strategies, and Risk-Free Support Products

PEYTON AUDREY

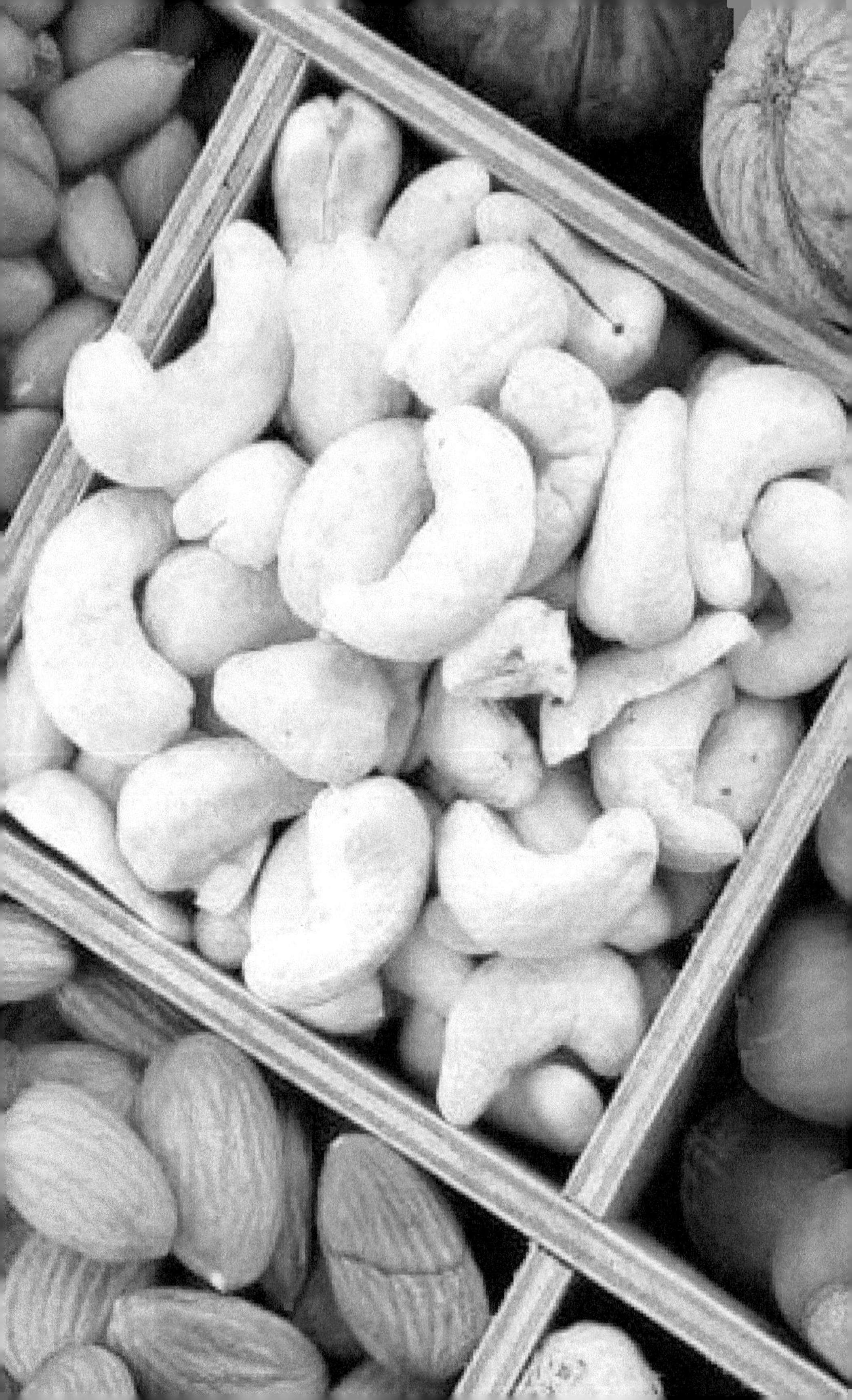

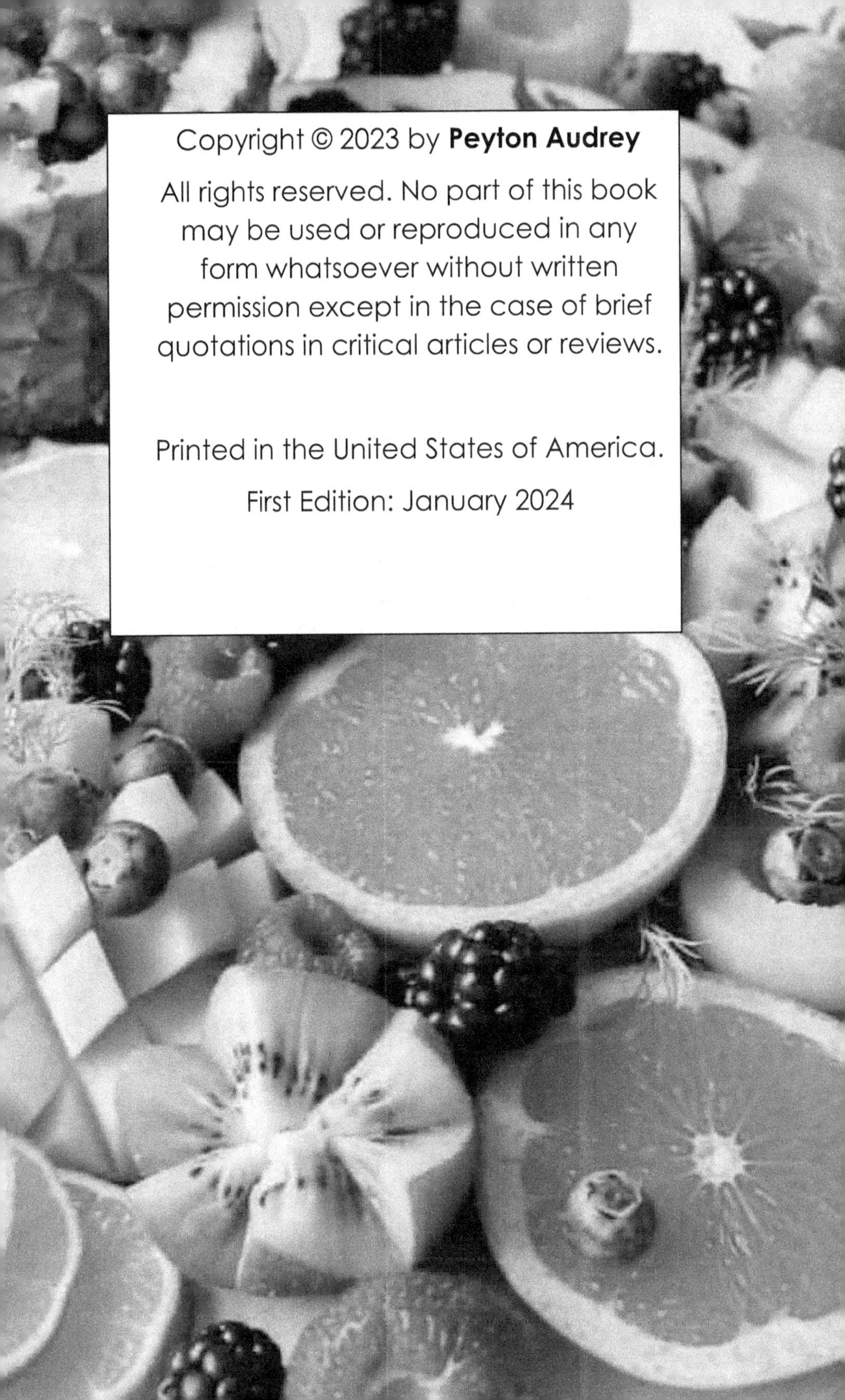

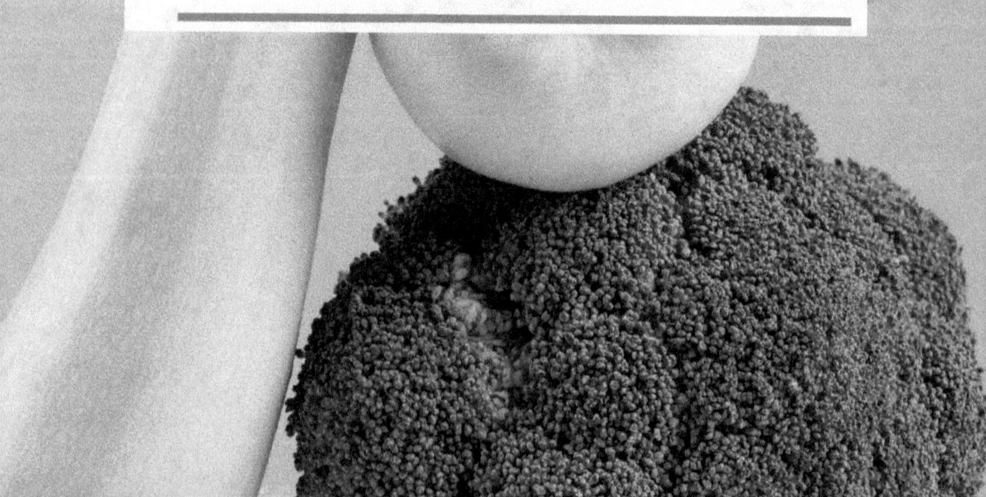

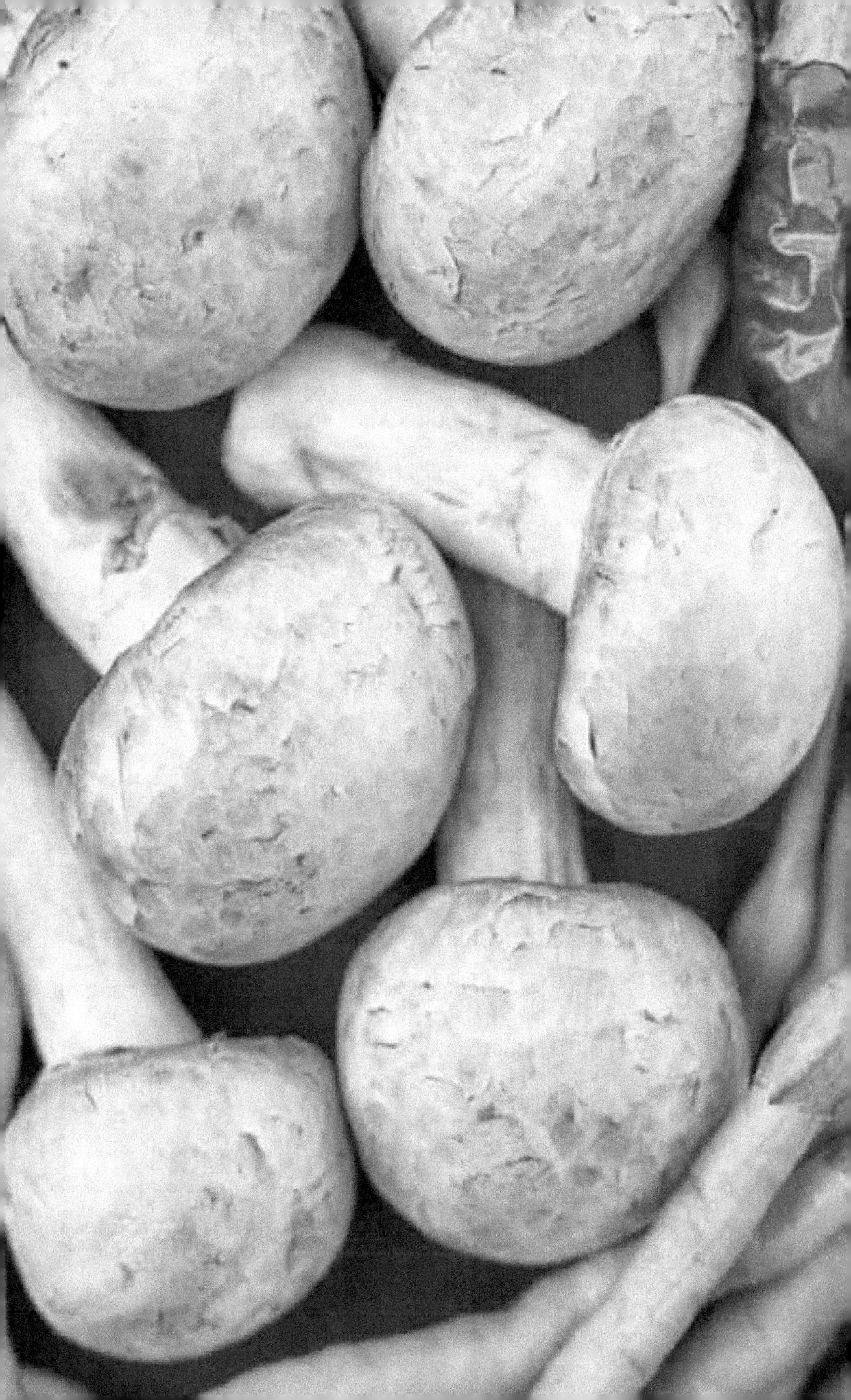

# TABLE OF CONTENT


**INTRODUCTION** .................................................................1

**Meet DEBBY James: A Personal** ..................................1

**Wellness Journey** ...............................................1

**Unveiling Peyton Audrey: Your Trusted Guide**........................4

**CHAPTER ONE** .................................................................7

**Understanding Hiatal Hernias After 40** ...........................7

**The Impact of Age on Hiatal Hernias** .............................7

**Common Symptoms and Challenges in Over 40s** ..................9

**Chapter two** ..................................................................12

**Holistic Approaches to Hiatal Hernia Management**..............12

**Peyton's Holistic Healing Strategies**...............................12

1. Mind-Body Connection: ......................................................12
2. Breathwork and Diaphragmatic Exercises: .........................12
3. Incorporating Physical Activity: .........................................13
4. Sleep Hygiene and Posture Awareness:..............................13
5. Emotional Well-being: .......................................................13
6. Individualized Dietary Guidance: .......................................14
7. Comprehensive Support:....................................................14

**Incorporating Mind, Body, and Soul into your Wellness Journey**......................................................................16

1. Mind:.................................................................................16
2. Body: ................................................................................16
3. Soul: .................................................................................17
Integration: ...........................................................................17

**CHAPTER THREE**.............................................................19

**Comprehensive Dietary Guidelines** ...................................**19**

**The Basics of Hiatal Hernia Diet: A Clear Understanding**.......**19**

**Long-Term Benefits of Making Dietary Changes**...................**22**

**CHAPTER FOUR** ...........................................................**25**

**Vegetarian and Organic Options**....................................**25**

**Embracing Plant-Based Nutrition**....................................**25**

**Recipes For Plant-Based Nutrition:**...................................**28**

Recipe 1: Rainbow Quinoa Salad ......................................28

Recipe 2: Chickpea and Vegetable Stir-Fry ........................29

Recipe 3: Ginger Turmeric Smoothie .................................31

Recipe 4: Baked Salmon with Lemon and Dill .....................31

Recipe 5: Quinoa and Vegetable Stir-Fry ...........................32

Recipe 6: Mango and Avocado Salad................................34

Recipe 7: Lentil and Vegetable Soup .................................35

Recipe 8: Baked Sweet Potato Fries ..................................36

Recipe 9: Chia Seed Pudding with Berries .........................37

Recipe 10: Minty Cucumber and Melon Salad .....................38

Recipe 11: Chickpea and Spinach Stew .............................39

Recipe 12: Baked Cod with Lemon Herb Crust .....................40

Recipe 13: Stuffed Bell Peppers with Quinoa and Black
Beans...........................................................................41

Recipe 14: Mango Ginger Chia Seed Pudding .....................42

Recipe 15: Lemon Basil Grilled Chicken ..............................43

Recipe 16: Turmeric Lentil Soup ........................................43

Recipe 17: Baked Herb-Crusted Turkey Breast......................44

Recipe 18: Spinach and Mushroom Quiche with Oat Crust..45

Recipe 19: Coconut Ginger Carrot Soup.............................46

Recipe 20: Buckwheat Banana Pancakes...........................47

**A One Week Meal Plan** ..................................................49

**The Delights of Organic and Gluten-Free Choices** .................52

**Recipes for Organic and Gluten-free choices:** ......................54

Recipe 1: Quinoa-Stuffed Bell Peppers .......................................54

Recipe 2: Organic Grilled Chicken Salad ...................................55

Recipe 3: Gluten-Free Zucchini Noodles with Pesto.............56

Recipe 4: Organic Berry Smoothie Bowl.................................57

Recipe 5: Gluten-Free Almond Flour Banana Bread.............58

Recipe 6: Organic Quinoa Salad with Lemon Vinaigrette ....59

Recipe 7: Gluten-Free Cauliflower Pizza Crust.......................60

Recipe 8: Organic Stir-Fried Tofu with Vegetables .................61

Recipe 9: Gluten-Free Almond Butter Banana Muffins .........62

Recipe 10: Organic Berry Chia Seed Popsicles ......................63

**Chapter five**....................................................................65

**Understanding Food Allergies**.............................................65

**and intolerance** ...............................................................65

**Dietary Allergies**...............................................................65

**Food Allergies** .................................................................68

Common Food Allergens:.......................................................68

Symptoms of Food Allergies: ..................................................69

Managing Food Allergies: ......................................................69

**CHAPTER SIX** ...................................................................73

**Convenience Meets Health: Snacks and Meal
Replacements**....................................................................73

**Healthy Snack Options for Busy Lifestyles**...........................73

**Meal Replacement Strategies for Sustainable Living**.............76

**CHAPTER SEVEN** ..............................................................79

Supportive Products for Hiatal Hernia.................................79

Hernia Belts and Truss Binders: An Overview .......................79

Hernia Belts:.............................................................................79

Features and Benefits: ............................................................79

Truss Binders: .........................................................................80

Features and Benefits: ............................................................80

Integration with hiatal hernia diet for over 40:....................80

Nature's Reveal: Vegetarian Capsules and Natural Dietary
Supplements ............................................................................82

Vegetarian Capsules:..............................................................82

Features and Benefits: ............................................................82

Natural Dietary Supplements: ................................................82

Key Components: ....................................................................83

Integration into hiatal hernia diet for over 40: ....................83

Chapter eight ..........................................................................85

Daily Activities and Fast Recovery Tips ................................85

Holistic Recovery: Integrating Daily Activities......................85

Tips For Fast Recovery and Overall Well-Being in Hiatal
Hernia Management.................................................................89

Chapter nine ...........................................................................93

Gender-Specific Support: Female...........................................93

Hernia Belt Design...................................................................93

Addressing Unique Needs for Women in Hiatal Hernia
Management .............................................................................93

Customized Support for Female Hiatal Hernia Patients .........97

**CHAPTER TEN**....................................................101

**Ensuring Optimum Elasticity:**.................................101

**Breathable Belt Features** ......................................101

**Understanding the Importance of Optimum Elasticity**.........101

**Lightweight Moisture-Wicking Fabric for Comfort** .............105

**Conclusion** ........................................................109

**Embrace Your Wellness Journey** ............................109

**Recap of Key Dietary and Lifestyle Strategies**.....................109

**Peyton Audrey's Encouragement for A Holistic Approach to Hiatal Hernia Management** ......................................113

# INTRODUCTION
# MEET DEBBY JAMES: A PERSONAL WELLNESS JOURNEY

In the quiet town of Amsterdam, nestled in the heart of New York, lived a 45-year-old business developer named Debby James. Debby, like many of us, found herself at a crossroads where health and daily life intersected in unexpected ways. Little did she know that her journey to wellness would be guided by an unexpected yet cherished friend, Peyton Audrey, a renowned dietitian and wellness expert.

Picture this: a cozy living room in Amsterdam, where the aroma of freshly brewed coffee wafts through the air as Debby and Peyton sit comfortably, engaged in a conversation that would redefine Debby's approach to health. As the evening sunbathes the room in warm hues, Peyton, with a warm smile, begins to unravel the secrets of the Hiatal Hernia Diet, not just as a set of recipes but as a transformative way of life.

Debby, having battled the discomforts of Hiatal Hernia for quite some time, felt an immediate connection with Peyton's approach. This was no ordinary journey Peyton was about to take Debby on; it was a journey that promised not just relief from symptoms but a revelation of a new, delicious, and sustainable way of living.

As Peyton delved into the basics of the Hiatal Hernia Diet, there were no complex terms or confusing medical jargon. It was like having a heart-to-heart chat with a dear friend who genuinely cared. Peyton shared stories, anecdotes, and real-life examples that resonated with Debby, making the seemingly daunting path of dietary changes feel like a natural progression.

The Hiatal Hernia Diet, Peyton explained, wasn't merely about managing a health condition; it was about taking charge of one's well-being. It was a lifestyle that promised more than just physical relief; it aimed for an emotional and mental equilibrium that would resonate in every aspect of Herley's life.

From the heart of Amsterdam to the bustling streets of New York, the journey unfolded. Peyton guided Debby through the intricacies of incorporating vegetarian and organic options into his daily meals. The aroma of gluten-free, GMO-free delights filled Debby's kitchen, and each bite brought her closer to a healthier version of herself.

Amid recipes and dietary advice, Peyton introduced Debby to a world where convenience met health. Squeeze packs of wholesome goodness became Debby's allies in her busy life, and the concept of meal replacements took on a whole new meaning. It wasn't just about the food on the plate; it was about nourishing the body, mind, and soul.

As the pages turned, and the journey continued, Peyton shared insights into the importance of support products like hernia belts and truss binders. It was a revelation for Debby, who discovered that holistic healing wasn't just about what she put into her body but also about the support and care she provided externally.

Join Debby on this extraordinary journey as she discovers the delights of vegetarian capsules, the harmony of natural dietary supplements, and the confidence that comes with a risk-free, satisfying experience. This isn't just a guide; it's a narrative of transformation, a tale of a friend leading another through the incredible world of the Hiatal Hernia Diet.

As you turn the pages of "Hiatal Hernia Diet for Over 40," envision yourself in Debby's shoes, walking alongside Peyton Audrey, your trusted friend and guide, towards a life where health and happiness intertwine seamlessly.

## UNVEILING PEYTON AUDREY: YOUR TRUSTED GUIDE

In the realm of wellness and dietary wisdom, there emerges a beacon of knowledge and compassion — Peyton Audrey. As we delve into the pages of "Hiatal Hernia Diet for Over 40," Peyton stands not just as a guide but as a trusted friend on your transformative journey.

**A Journey of Expertise:** Peyton Audrey is no stranger to the intricacies of nutrition and holistic well-being. With a background steeped in dietetics and a passion for empowering individuals, Peyton brings a wealth of knowledge to the table. Herley James, a 45-year-old business developer from Amsterdam, New York, found solace and guidance in Peyton's expertise during his own Hiatal Hernia journey.

**Compassion in Every Word:** What sets Peyton apart is not just the depth of professional knowledge, but the genuine compassion woven into every piece of advice. As you turn the pages, you'll sense a guiding hand that understands the struggles, the uncertainties, and the hopes that accompany the path to wellness. Peyton's approach is like that of a caring friend, ensuring that no aspect of your well-being is left unattended.

**Holistic Healing Advocate:** Peyton Audrey advocates not merely for a dietary change but for a holistic shift in lifestyle. Her insights transcend the plate, delving into the interconnectedness of mind, body, and soul. This holistic approach ensures that your journey toward managing Hiatal Hernia is not just about symptom relief but about embracing a life of vitality and balance.

**Tailored Guidance for All:** Whether you are a seasoned wellness enthusiast or taking your first steps toward a healthier lifestyle, Peyton's guidance is tailored for all. The clarity with which complex concepts are unravelled makes Peyton's expertise accessible and relatable. No question is too small, no concern too trivial — Peyton's commitment to your well-being shines through in every interaction.

**A Trusted Companion:** As you navigate the nuances of the Hiatal Hernia Diet, Peyton Audrey becomes more than an expert — she becomes a trusted companion. Through discussions on dietary guidelines, vegetarian and organic options, supportive products, and daily activities, Peyton's voice resonates as that of a friend leading you toward a life of vibrancy and resilience.

In "Hiatal Hernia Diet for Over 40," Peyton Audrey opens the door to a world where health, happiness, and holistic well-being converge. Join us on this journey as Peyton, your trusted guide, unravels the secrets of a fulfilling and sustainable life. The pages are not just filled with information; they are imbued with the warmth of a friend's understanding and the expertise of a dedicated wellness advocate. Embrace Peyton Audrey's guidance, and let the transformation begin.

## CHAPTER ONE
## UNDERSTANDING HIATAL HERNIAS AFTER 40

## THE IMPACT OF AGE ON HIATAL HERNIAS

"The Impact of Age on Hiatal Hernias" refers to the influence that advancing age can have on the development, symptoms, and management of hiatal hernias. A hiatal hernia occurs when part of the stomach protrudes through the diaphragm into the chest cavity, and various factors, including age, can contribute to its occurrence.

As individuals age, several physiological changes in the body may increase the likelihood of hiatal hernias. These changes can include a weakening of the muscles and tissues that support the diaphragm and the lower esophageal sphincter (LES), which is a muscular ring that separates the esophagus from the stomach.

The impact of age on hiatal hernias may manifest in several ways:

1. **Weakening of Muscles:** Aging can lead to a natural weakening of muscles, including those around the diaphragm. This weakening may contribute to the formation or exacerbation of hiatal hernias.

2. **Increased Pressure in the Abdomen:** Factors such as obesity, which may become more prevalent with age, can lead to increased pressure in the abdominal cavity. This pressure can contribute to the stomach pushing through the weakened diaphragm.

3. **Changes in Connective Tissues:** The connective tissues that provide support to the organs and structures in the abdominal region may undergo

changes with age, potentially affecting their ability to keep the stomach in its proper position.

4. **Reduced Esophageal Sphincter Tone:** The LES, a circular muscle that separates the esophagus from the stomach, may experience a decline in tone with age. This reduced tone can contribute to the reflux of stomach contents into the esophagus.

Understanding the impact of age on hiatal hernias is crucial for individuals over 40, as it sheds light on why they may be more susceptible to developing or experiencing complications related to hiatal hernias. It underscores the importance of adopting lifestyle and dietary practices that can mitigate these age-related factors and promote overall digestive health. Additionally, it emphasizes the need for tailored approaches to managing hiatal hernias in different age groups, taking into account the specific challenges that may arise with advancing age.

# COMMON SYMPTOMS AND CHALLENGES IN OVER 40S

As individuals enter their 40s and beyond, they may experience common symptoms and challenges related to hiatal hernias, a condition where part of the stomach protrudes into the chest cavity through the diaphragm. Understanding these symptoms and challenges is crucial for identifying and managing hiatal hernias in individuals over 40. Here's a detailed exploration:

1. **Reflux and Heartburn:**

   - **Symptoms:** Over 40s with hiatal hernias often experience frequent heartburn and acid reflux. The protrusion of the stomach through the diaphragm can weaken the lower esophageal sphincter (LES), allowing stomach acid to flow into the esophagus, leading to discomfort and a burning sensation.

   - **Challenges:** Persistent reflux can contribute to esophagitis (inflammation of the esophagus) and increase the risk of developing conditions like Barrett's esophagus.

2. **Difficulty Swallowing (Dysphagia):**

   - **Symptoms:** Hiatal hernias may cause difficulty swallowing, especially when the herniated portion of the stomach obstructs the normal passage of food through the esophagus.

   - **Challenges:** Dysphagia can lead to inadequate nutrition and weight loss if not addressed. It may also impact the overall quality of life by affecting the enjoyment of meals.

## 3. Chest Pain and Discomfort:

- **Symptoms:** Some individuals with hiatal hernias experience chest pain and discomfort, which can be mistaken for cardiac issues. This pain may be exacerbated after meals or when lying down.

- **Challenges:** Distinguishing between hiatal hernia-related chest pain and cardiac-related chest pain is crucial. Seeking medical attention for chest pain is imperative to rule out serious conditions.

## 4. Regurgitation:

- **Symptoms:** Over 40s with hiatal hernias may regurgitate stomach contents into the mouth, leading to a sour taste and the sensation of fluid backing up into the throat.

- **Challenges:** Regurgitation can contribute to dental issues due to exposure of tooth enamel to stomach acid. It may also lead to throat irritation and chronic cough.

## 5. Respiratory Issues:

- **Symptoms:** Hiatal hernias can cause respiratory symptoms such as chronic cough, wheezing, or asthma-like symptoms due to the irritation of the airways by stomach acid.

- **Challenges:** Respiratory symptoms may be challenging to diagnose correctly, requiring a comprehensive evaluation to differentiate between hiatal hernia-related issues and other respiratory conditions.

## 6. Anemia and Fatigue:

- **Symptoms:** Chronic bleeding from the irritation of the esophagus by stomach acid may lead to anemia, resulting in fatigue and weakness.

- **Challenges:** Identifying and addressing anemia is crucial to prevent complications and improve overall well-being.

## 7. Increased Risk of Complications:

- **Symptoms:** Individuals over 40 with hiatal hernias may face an increased risk of complications such as esophageal strictures, ulcers, and in severe cases, Barrett's esophagus.

- **Challenges:** Regular monitoring and management are essential to prevent the progression of hiatal hernia-related complications.

Understanding these symptoms and challenges empowers individuals over 40 to seek timely medical attention, adopt lifestyle modifications, and work with healthcare professionals to manage hiatal hernias effectively. Early intervention can alleviate symptoms, improve quality of life, and prevent the progression of complications associated with hiatal hernias.

# CHAPTER TWO
# HOLISTIC APPROACHES TO HIATAL HERNIA MANAGEMENT

## PEYTON'S HOLISTIC HEALING STRATEGIES

"Peyton's Holistic Healing Strategies" encompass a multifaceted approach to managing hiatal hernias in individuals over 40, acknowledging that a comprehensive strategy goes beyond dietary changes alone. Here's a balanced and detailed exploration of Peyton's holistic healing strategies in the context of "Hiatal Hernia Diet for Over 40":

### 1. Mind-Body Connection:

- ***Explanation:*** Peyton recognizes the profound connection between the mind and body in achieving overall well-being. Stress and anxiety can exacerbate symptoms of hiatal hernias. Therefore, Peyton encourages practices such as mindfulness, meditation, and stress-reducing activities to foster emotional balance.

- ***Relevance:*** Stress management is crucial in preventing the exacerbation of symptoms related to hiatal hernias, as stress can influence digestive processes and contribute to reflux.

### 2. Breathwork and Diaphragmatic Exercises:

- ***Explanation:*** Peyton introduces breathwork and diaphragmatic exercises as integral components of holistic healing. Strengthening the diaphragm can provide better support to the lower esophageal sphincter, reducing the likelihood of stomach protrusion.

- **_Relevance:_** Diaphragmatic exercises enhance diaphragm function, potentially mitigating the impact of hiatal hernias by fortifying the natural barrier between the abdomen and chest.

## 3. Incorporating Physical Activity:

- **_Explanation:_** Peyton advocates for regular physical activity tailored to individual capabilities. Exercise promotes overall health, helps maintain a healthy weight, and contributes to optimal digestive function.

- **_Relevance:_** Physical activity is associated with improved digestion and can assist in weight management, addressing factors that may contribute to hiatal hernia development or exacerbation.

## 4. Sleep Hygiene and Posture Awareness:

- **_Explanation:_** Peyton emphasizes the importance of good sleep hygiene and posture awareness. Maintaining an elevated upper body position during sleep can help prevent acid reflux, reducing the likelihood of nighttime symptoms.

- **_Relevance:_** Adequate sleep and proper posture contribute to overall health and can specifically alleviate symptoms associated with hiatal hernias, such as reflux and discomfort.

## 5. Emotional Well-being:

- **_Explanation:_** Peyton addresses the emotional aspects of living with a chronic condition. Providing guidance on navigating emotional challenges and offering a supportive approach is integral to the holistic healing process.

- ***Relevance:*** Emotional well-being is interconnected with physical health. Addressing emotional aspects contributes to an individual's overall resilience and coping mechanisms in managing hiatal hernias.

## 6. Individualized Dietary Guidance:

- ***Explanation:*** Peyton tailors dietary guidance to individual needs, incorporating elements such as vegetarian and organic options, gluten-free choices, and convenient yet health-conscious snacks.

- ***Relevance:*** Dietary modifications form a cornerstone of hiatal hernia management. Peyton's approach considers the diverse dietary preferences and restrictions of individuals over 40, ensuring that the recommended changes are practical and sustainable.

## 7. Comprehensive Support:

- ***Explanation:*** Peyton advocates for a holistic support system that includes dietary changes, lifestyle adjustments, and emotional well-being. The combination of these elements contributes to a more resilient and balanced approach to hiatal hernia management.

- ***Relevance:*** Recognizing that holistic healing involves multiple facets, Peyton's strategies provide individuals over 40 with a well-rounded approach to managing hiatal hernias, addressing not only symptoms but also contributing factors and overall health.

In summary, Peyton's holistic healing strategies recognize the interconnectedness of physical, emotional, and lifestyle factors in the context of managing hiatal hernias in individuals over 40. By incorporating mindfulness, breathwork, physical activity, sleep hygiene, emotional well-being, and individualized dietary guidance, Peyton offers a comprehensive approach that empowers individuals to actively participate in their well-being journey.

15

## Incorporating Mind, Body, and Soul into your Wellness Journey

"Incorporating Mind, Body, and Soul into Your Wellness Journey" underscores the holistic approach to health and well-being, recognizing that an individual's overall wellness is interconnected with the well-being of their mind, body, and soul. Let's delve into an explanation of how this integration works:

1. Mind:

- **Explanation:** The mind plays a pivotal role in overall health, influencing both mental and physical well-being. Incorporating the mind into your wellness journey involves practices such as mindfulness, meditation, and stress reduction techniques. By cultivating a positive mindset and managing stress, individuals can positively impact their mental health, leading to a cascade of benefits for the body and soul.

- **Relevance:** Stress is known to exacerbate symptoms of conditions like hiatal hernias. By incorporating practices that nurture mental well-being, individuals can reduce stress levels, potentially alleviating symptoms and contributing to overall health.

2. Body:

- **Explanation:** The body is the physical vessel that carries us through life. Incorporating the body into your wellness journey involves adopting healthy lifestyle practices, including regular exercise, balanced nutrition, and adequate sleep. Physical activity supports digestive health, helps maintain a healthy weight, and contributes to overall vitality.

- **_Relevance:_** In the context of hiatal hernia management, strengthening the body through appropriate exercises, maintaining a healthy weight, and adopting dietary changes are essential components. These actions contribute not only to symptom relief but also to the prevention of further complications.

## 3. Soul:

- **_Explanation:_** The soul represents the essence of an individual — their innermost self. Nurturing the soul involves activities that bring joy, fulfillment, and a sense of purpose. This can include hobbies, creative pursuits, spending time in nature, or engaging in spiritual practices.

- **_Relevance:_** The emotional and spiritual well-being of an individual is integral to holistic health. Living with a chronic condition like a hiatal hernia may present emotional challenges. Nurturing the soul by engaging in activities that bring joy and meaning can enhance resilience and contribute to an individual's ability to cope with health challenges.

## Integration:

- **_Explanation:_** True holistic wellness involves the integration of mind, body, and soul. It's about recognizing the synergy between these elements and fostering a balanced and harmonious existence. For example, adopting a mindful eating practice (mind) contributes to both physical health by aiding digestion and emotional well-being by fostering a positive relationship with food.

- **_Relevance:_** In the context of hiatal hernia management, this integrated approach ensures that individuals not only address physical symptoms but also attend to the emotional and spiritual aspects of their well-being. This comprehensive strategy contributes to a more resilient and sustainable wellness journey.

By incorporating mind, body, and soul into the wellness journey, individuals can cultivate a state of balance that extends beyond symptom management. It's about fostering a lifestyle that supports overall health and resilience, recognizing that true well-being involves a harmonious relationship between mental, physical, and spiritual aspects of our being.

## THE BASICS OF HIATAL HERNIA DIET: A CLEAR UNDERSTANDING

"The Basics of Hiatal Hernia Diet: A Clear Understanding" involves breaking down the fundamental principles of dietary management for individuals with hiatal hernias. Let's explore this concept in detail:

### 1. Understanding the Condition:

- ***Explanation:*** Before delving into the specifics of a hiatal hernia diet, it's crucial to have a clear understanding of the condition itself. A hiatal hernia occurs when part of the stomach pushes through the diaphragm into the chest cavity. This displacement can lead to symptoms such as acid reflux, heartburn, and difficulty swallowing.

- ***Relevance:*** A clear comprehension of the condition lays the foundation for dietary choices. Understanding how the anatomy is affected helps individuals make informed decisions about the types of foods that may exacerbate or alleviate symptoms.

### 2. Importance of Lowering Acidic Foods:

- ***Explanation:*** One of the key principles of a hiatal hernia diet involves reducing the intake of acidic foods. Stomach acid can easily flow back into the esophagus through the weakened lower esophageal sphincter (LES). Limiting acidic foods helps minimize the risk of acid reflux and irritation of the esophagus.

- **Relevance:** Lowering acidic food intake is essential for managing symptoms such as heartburn and regurgitation, common in individuals with hiatal hernias.

## 3. Emphasizing Non-Acidic, Alkaline Foods:

- **Explanation:** On the flip side, a hiatal hernia diet encourages the consumption of non-acidic, alkaline foods. These include fruits and vegetables with a low acidity level, promoting a more alkaline environment in the stomach. Alkaline foods are less likely to trigger reflux.

- **Relevance:** Incorporating alkaline foods into the diet helps create a more favorable environment, reducing the likelihood of stomach acid irritating the esophagus.

## 4. Mindful Eating and Portion Control:

- **Explanation:** Mindful eating involves paying attention to the act of eating and being aware of the sensations and flavors. Additionally, practicing portion control can prevent overeating, which can put pressure on the stomach and contribute to reflux.

- **Relevance:** Mindful eating and portion control are crucial aspects of a hiatal hernia diet, promoting digestive comfort and minimizing symptoms.

## 5. Avoiding Trigger Foods:

- **Explanation:** Identifying and avoiding trigger foods is an essential component of a hiatal hernia diet. These are foods that can worsen symptoms, such as spicy foods, caffeine, chocolate, and fatty foods.

- **Relevance:** Steering clear of trigger foods helps individuals manage symptoms effectively and prevent the recurrence of discomfort associated with hiatal hernias.

## 6. Incorporating Fiber-Rich Foods:

- **Explanation:** Including fiber-rich foods in the diet, such as whole grains, fruits, and vegetables, supports digestive health. Fiber aids in regular bowel movements and can prevent constipation, a common concern for individuals with hiatal hernias.

- **Relevance:** Maintaining good digestive health is important in managing overall well-being and minimizing complications associated with hiatal hernias.

## 7. Hydration and Timing of Meals:

- **Explanation:** Staying adequately hydrated and being mindful of the timing of meals are integral to a hiatal hernia diet. Drinking water between meals, rather than during, can prevent the stomach from becoming overly full and reduce the risk of reflux.

- **Relevance:** Proper hydration and strategic meal timing contribute to a comfortable digestive experience, minimizing the likelihood of symptoms.

In essence, the basics of a hiatal hernia diet involve a thoughtful and informed approach to food choices. Understanding the condition, focusing on lower acidity, incorporating alkaline foods, practicing mindful eating, avoiding triggers, including fiber, and being mindful of hydration and meal timing collectively form a dietary strategy aimed at managing symptoms and promoting overall digestive well-being.

## Long-Term Benefits of Making Dietary Changes

For individuals with hiatal hernias extend beyond immediate symptom relief and contribute to overall health and well-being. Let's explore the lasting advantages of adopting a hiatal hernia-friendly diet over the long term:

### 1. Reduced Symptom Severity:

- *Explanation:* Consistent adherence to a hiatal hernia-friendly diet can lead to a significant reduction in the severity and frequency of symptoms such as acid reflux, heartburn, and regurgitation.

- *Long-term Benefit:* By minimizing symptom severity, individuals experience improved comfort and quality of life over an extended period.

### 2. Prevention of Complications:

- *Explanation:* Long-term adherence to dietary changes helps prevent complications associated with hiatal hernias, such as esophagitis, Barrett's esophagus, and strictures.

- *Long-term Benefit:* Prevention of complications contributes to overall health and reduces the risk of developing more serious conditions related to untreated hiatal hernias.

### 3. Weight Management:

- *Explanation:* Adopting a hiatal hernia-friendly diet often involves making choices that support weight management, such as portion control and choosing nutrient-dense foods.

- *Long-term Benefit:* Maintaining a healthy weight over the long term not only supports digestive health but also contributes to overall well-being and reduces the strain on the lower esophageal sphincter.

## 4. Improved Nutrient Absorption:

- **Explanation:** A well-balanced hiatal hernia diet, rich in fiber and essential nutrients, supports optimal nutrient absorption in the digestive system.

- **Long-term Benefit:** Improved nutrient absorption contributes to overall health, energy levels, and the body's ability to function optimally.

## 5. Enhanced Digestive Comfort:

- **Explanation:** Dietary changes that focus on avoiding trigger foods, promoting mindful eating, and incorporating fiber-rich options contribute to enhanced digestive comfort.

- **Long-term Benefit:** Individuals experience sustained relief from discomfort, promoting a positive and comfortable daily digestive experience.

## 6. Prevention of Acid-related Dental Issues:

- **Explanation:** Long-term adherence to a hiatal hernia-friendly diet helps prevent acid-related dental problems, such as enamel erosion and tooth decay.

- **Long-term Benefit:** Protecting dental health contributes to overall well-being and prevents the need for extensive dental interventions.

## 7. Sustainable Lifestyle Habits:

- **Explanation:** Adopting a hiatal hernia-friendly diet often involves cultivating sustainable lifestyle habits, such as mindful eating, portion control, and regular physical activity.

- **Long-term Benefit:** Sustainable habits contribute to overall health and longevity, providing individuals with tools for maintaining well-being throughout their lives.

## 8. Emotional Well-being:

- ***Explanation:*** Long-term adherence to dietary changes supports emotional well-being by reducing the impact of symptoms on mental health and fostering a positive relationship with food.

- ***Long-term Benefit:*** Emotional well-being is a key component of overall health, and a positive mindset can contribute to resilience in managing the challenges associated with a chronic condition like a hiatal hernia.

In summary, the long-term benefits of making dietary changes for individuals with hiatal hernias go beyond managing immediate symptoms. By adopting a sustainable, hiatal hernia-friendly diet, individuals can experience lasting improvements in digestive health, prevent complications, and promote overall well-being over the course of their lives.

# CHAPTER FOUR
# VEGETARIAN AND ORGANIC OPTIONS

## EMBRACING PLANT-BASED NUTRITION

Involves prioritizing and incorporating a wide variety of plant-derived foods into one's diet. This dietary approach emphasizes fruits, vegetables, whole grains, legumes, nuts, and seeds, while minimizing or excluding animal products. Let's delve into a more detailed exploration of the concept:

1. **Incorporating a Colorful Array of Vegetables and Fruits:**

   - ***Explanation:*** Plant-based nutrition encourages the consumption of a diverse range of colorful vegetables and fruits. These foods are rich in vitamins, minerals, antioxidants, and fiber, contributing to overall health.

   - ***Benefits:*** The varied nutrients in vegetables and fruits support immune function, provide essential vitamins, and help maintain digestive health, factors crucial for individuals managing hiatal hernias.

2. **Whole Grains as Dietary Staples:**

   - ***Explanation:*** Plant-based diets emphasize whole grains like brown rice, quinoa, oats, and whole wheat. Whole grains are a valuable source of complex carbohydrates and fiber, promoting sustained energy and digestive health.

   - ***Benefits:*** The fiber content in whole grains aids in digestion, helps prevent constipation, and supports overall gut health, factors relevant to individuals seeking comfort in managing hiatal hernias.

3. **Legumes as Protein Sources:**

- *Explanation:* Plant-based nutrition often includes legumes such as beans, lentils, and chickpeas as primary protein sources. Legumes are not only rich in protein but also provide essential nutrients like iron and fiber.

- *Benefits:* Legumes offer a plant-based protein alternative that is lower in fat and can contribute to a feeling of fullness, supporting weight management—a consideration for individuals with hiatal hernias.

4. **Nuts and Seeds for Healthy Fats:**

- *Explanation:* Plant-based diets incorporate nuts and seeds for healthy fats, including omega-3 fatty acids. These fats support cardiovascular health and provide a nutrient-dense source of energy.

- *Benefits:* Healthy fats from nuts and seeds contribute to overall well-being and can be a valuable component of a hiatal hernia-friendly diet, considering their nutrient profile and potential to aid in weight management.

5. **Minimizing or Eliminating Animal Products:**

- *Explanation:* Embracing plant-based nutrition involves minimizing or eliminating the intake of animal products such as meat, dairy, and eggs. This choice aligns with the goal of deriving most nutrients from plant sources.

- *Benefits:* A plant-based approach may reduce saturated fat intake and contribute to better heart health. Additionally, some individuals with hiatal hernias find that minimizing certain animal products helps alleviate symptoms like acid reflux.

## 6. **Promoting Digestive Health with Fiber:**

- ***Explanation:*** Plant-based diets, rich in fruits, vegetables, and whole grains, naturally provide ample dietary fiber. Fiber supports digestive health by promoting regular bowel movements and preventing constipation.

- ***Benefits:*** For individuals with hiatal hernias, maintaining regular bowel movements can contribute to overall digestive comfort and reduce the risk of complications associated with constipation.

## 7. **Diversity in Nutrient Intake:**

- ***Explanation:*** Plant-based nutrition encourages a diverse intake of nutrients from a wide array of plant sources. This diversity ensures a broad spectrum of vitamins, minerals, and antioxidants.

- ***Benefits:*** A varied nutrient intake supports overall health and can be particularly beneficial for individuals managing hiatal hernias, helping meet nutritional needs without relying heavily on potentially triggering foods.

In summary, embracing plant-based nutrition involves a conscientious choice to center one's diet around plant-derived foods. This dietary approach offers a wealth of nutritional benefits, supporting overall health and potentially providing relief for individuals managing hiatal hernias. However, it's important to approach any dietary changes with consideration for individual needs and preferences, consulting with healthcare professionals as necessary.

## RECIPES FOR PLANT-BASED NUTRITION:

Here are twenty nutrient-rich plant-based recipes that align with the principles of "Embracing Plant-Based Nutrition." Each recipe is designed to contribute to overall health and provide potential benefits for individuals managing hiatal hernias.

Recipe 1: Rainbow Quinoa Salad

**Ingredients:**

- 1 cup quinoa (rainbow or regular)
- 2 cups water
- 1 cup cherry tomatoes, halved
- 1 cucumber, diced
- 1 bell pepper (red or yellow), diced
- 1 cup shredded carrots
- 1/2 cup red onion, finely chopped
- 1/4 cup fresh parsley, chopped
- 1/4 cup extra-virgin olive oil
- 2 tablespoons balsamic vinegar
- Salt and pepper to taste
- **Optional:** Avocado slices for serving

**Instructions:**

1. Rinse the quinoa thoroughly. In a saucepan, combine quinoa and water. Bring to a boil, then reduce heat to low, cover, and simmer for 15-20 minutes or until quinoa is cooked and water is absorbed. Let it cool.

2. In a large bowl, combine cooled quinoa, cherry tomatoes, cucumber, bell pepper, shredded carrots, red onion, and fresh parsley.

3. In a small bowl, whisk together olive oil, balsamic vinegar, salt, and pepper.

4. Pour the dressing over the salad and toss until well combined.

5. Serve in bowls, and garnish with avocado slices if desired.

## Nutritional Facts and Why It's Nutrient-Rich:

- Quinoa is a complete protein, providing all essential amino acids.

- Colorful vegetables offer a variety of vitamins, minerals, and antioxidants.

- Olive oil provides healthy monounsaturated fats.

- Avocado adds heart-healthy fats and creaminess.

- High fiber content supports digestive health.

## Recipe 2: Chickpea and Vegetable Stir-Fry

## Ingredients:

- 1 can (15 oz) chickpeas, drained and rinsed

- 2 cups broccoli florets

- 1 bell pepper (any color), sliced

- 1 cup snap peas, ends trimmed

- 1 carrot, julienned

- 3 cloves garlic, minced

- 1 tablespoon ginger, grated

- 3 tablespoons soy sauce (or tamari for a gluten-free option)

- 1 tablespoon sesame oil

- 1 tablespoon maple syrup or agave nectar

- 2 tablespoons sesame seeds (optional)

- Brown rice or quinoa for serving

**Instructions:**

1. In a large skillet or wok, heat sesame oil over medium-high heat. Add garlic and ginger, sauté for 1-2 minutes until fragrant.

2. Add broccoli, bell pepper, snap peas, and carrot to the skillet. Stir-fry for 5-7 minutes until vegetables are tender-crisp.

3. Add chickpeas to the vegetables and stir to combine.

4. In a small bowl, whisk together soy sauce and maple syrup. Pour the sauce over the stir-fry and toss until everything is well coated.

5. Serve the stir-fry over brown rice or quinoa, and sprinkle with sesame seeds if desired.

**Nutritional Facts and Why It's Nutrient-Rich:**

- Chickpeas provide plant-based protein and fiber.

- Colorful vegetables offer vitamins, minerals, and antioxidants.

- Ginger and garlic have anti-inflammatory properties.

- Sesame oil adds healthy fats.

- Whole grains contribute additional fiber for digestive health.

## Ingredients:

- 1 cup fresh pineapple chunks
- 1 banana
- 1/2 teaspoon grated ginger
- 1/2 teaspoon ground turmeric
- 1 cup coconut water
- Ice cubes (optional)

## Instructions:

1. Combine pineapple, banana, grated ginger, ground turmeric, and coconut water in a blender.
2. Blend until smooth.
3. Add ice cubes if desired and blend again.
4. Pour into a glass and enjoy!

## Nutritional Information:

- Rich in anti-inflammatory compounds from ginger and turmeric.
- Pineapple provides digestive enzymes, aiding in digestion.
- Banana adds potassium and natural sweetness.
- Coconut water hydrates and provides electrolytes.

## Recipe 4: Baked Salmon with Lemon and Dill

## Ingredients:

- 4 salmon fillets
- 1 lemon, sliced
- 2 tablespoons fresh dill, chopped

- 2 tablespoons olive oil

- Salt and pepper to taste

## Instructions:

1. Preheat the oven to 375°F (190°C).

2. Place salmon fillets on a baking sheet.

3. Drizzle with olive oil and season with salt and pepper.

4. Top each fillet with lemon slices and sprinkle with fresh dill.

5. Bake for 15-20 minutes or until the salmon is cooked through.

6. Serve with steamed vegetables or a side salad.

## Nutritional Information:

- Salmon is a good source of omega-3 fatty acids, supporting heart and digestive health.

- Lemon provides a burst of vitamin C and adds a refreshing flavor.

- Dill adds flavor without triggering acidity.

## Recipe 5: Quinoa and Vegetable Stir-Fry

## Ingredients:

- 1 cup quinoa

- 2 cups broccoli florets

- 1 bell pepper (any color), sliced

- 1 cup snap peas, ends trimmed

- 2 carrots, julienned

- 3 cloves garlic, minced

- 2 tablespoons low-sodium soy sauce

- 1 tablespoon sesame oil

- 1 tablespoon rice vinegar

**Instructions:**

1. Rinse quinoa and cook according to package instructions.

2. In a large skillet, heat sesame oil over medium-high heat.

3. Add garlic, broccoli, bell pepper, snap peas, and carrots. Stir-fry for 5-7 minutes until vegetables are tender-crisp.

4. Add cooked quinoa to the skillet.

5. In a small bowl, whisk together soy sauce and rice vinegar. Pour over the quinoa and vegetables, tossing to combine.

6. Serve immediately.

**Nutritional Information:**

- Quinoa provides a complete protein source.

- Colorful vegetables offer a range of vitamins and minerals.

- Sesame oil adds healthy fats.

- Soy sauce contributes umami flavor with reduced sodium.

## Ingredients:

- 2 cups mixed salad greens
- 1 ripe mango, diced
- 1 avocado, diced
- 1/4 cup red onion, thinly sliced
- 2 tablespoons chopped fresh cilantro
- Juice of 1 lime
- 1 tablespoon extra-virgin olive oil
- Salt and pepper to taste

## Instructions:

1. In a large bowl, combine salad greens, diced mango, diced avocado, red onion, and cilantro.
2. In a small bowl, whisk together lime juice, olive oil, salt, and pepper.
3. Drizzle the dressing over the salad and toss gently to combine.
4. Serve immediately.

## Nutritional Information:

- Mango and avocado provide vitamins and healthy fats.
- Mixed greens offer fiber and essential nutrients.
- Lime juice adds a burst of flavor without acidity.

# Recipe 7: Lentil and Vegetable Soup

## Ingredients:

- 1 cup dried green or brown lentils, rinsed
- 1 onion, diced
- 2 carrots, diced
- 2 celery stalks, diced
- 3 cloves garlic, minced
- 1 teaspoon ground cumin
- 1 teaspoon ground coriander
- 6 cups vegetable broth
- 1 can (14 oz) diced tomatoes
- Salt and pepper to taste
- Fresh parsley for garnish

## Instructions:

1. In a large pot, sauté onions, carrots, and celery until softened.
2. Add garlic, ground cumin, and ground coriander. Stir for 1-2 minutes.
3. Add lentils, vegetable broth, and diced tomatoes with their juices.
4. Bring to a boil, then reduce heat and simmer for 25-30 minutes until lentils are tender.
5. Season with salt and pepper to taste.
6. Garnish with fresh parsley before serving.

**Nutritional Information:**

- Lentils provide plant-based protein and fiber.

- Vegetables offer vitamins and minerals.

- Cumin and coriander add flavor without triggering acidity.

### Recipe 8: Baked Sweet Potato Fries

**Ingredients:**

- 2 large sweet potatoes, cut into fries

- 2 tablespoons olive oil

- 1 teaspoon smoked paprika

- 1/2 teaspoon garlic powder

- 1/2 teaspoon onion powder

- Salt and pepper to taste

**Instructions:**

1. Preheat the oven to 425°F (220°C).

2. In a large bowl, toss sweet potato fries with olive oil, smoked paprika, garlic powder, onion powder, salt, and pepper.

3. Spread the fries in a single layer on a baking sheet.

4. Bake for 25-30 minutes, flipping halfway through, until fries are golden and crisp.

5. Serve with a side of hummus or a plant-based dip.

**Nutritional Information:**

- Sweet potatoes are rich in vitamins, fiber, and antioxidants.

- Olive oil adds healthy fats.

- Smoked paprika provides flavor without acidity.



## Ingredients:

- 1/4 cup chia seeds
- 1 cup almond milk (or any plant-based milk)
- 1 tablespoon maple syrup or agave nectar
- 1/2 teaspoon vanilla extract
- Mixed berries for topping

## Instructions:

1. In a bowl, whisk together chia seeds, almond milk, maple syrup, and vanilla extract.
2. Cover and refrigerate for at least 2 hours or overnight, allowing the chia seeds to absorb the liquid and create a pudding-like consistency.
3. Stir the pudding before serving.
4. Top with mixed berries before serving.

## Nutritional Information:

- Chia seeds provide omega-3 fatty acids and fiber.
- Almond milk is a plant-based alternative rich in vitamins.
- Berries offer antioxidants and natural sweetness.

## Why They're Nutrient-Rich:

- **Balanced Macronutrients:** Each recipe incorporates a balance of carbohydrates, proteins, and healthy fats to support overall health and digestion.
- **Fiber Content:** Fiber-rich ingredients contribute to digestive comfort and regular bowel movements.

- **Anti-Inflammatory Ingredients:** Recipes include ingredients with anti-inflammatory properties to reduce irritation and discomfort.

- **Vitamins and Minerals:** Colorful fruits and vegetables provide essential vitamins and minerals for overall well-being.

- **Plant-Based Protein:** Plant-based protein sources such as lentils and quinoa support muscle health without contributing to acid reflux.

### Recipe 10: Minty Cucumber and Melon Salad

**Ingredients:**

- 2 cups diced cucumber

- 2 cups diced honeydew melon

- 1/4 cup fresh mint leaves, chopped

- 1 tablespoon lime juice

- 1 teaspoon honey

- Pinch of salt

**Instructions:**

1. In a large bowl, combine diced cucumber and honeydew melon.

2. In a small bowl, whisk together lime juice, honey, and a pinch of salt.

3. Pour the dressing over the salad and toss gently.

4. Chill in the refrigerator for 30 minutes before serving.

## Nutritional Information:

- Cucumber and melon provide hydration and are gentle on the stomach.

- Mint aids digestion and adds a refreshing flavor.

- Lime juice adds a burst of vitamin C without acidity.

## Recipe 11: Chickpea and Spinach Stew

## Ingredients:

- 1 can (15 oz) chickpeas, drained and rinsed

- 1 onion, chopped

- 2 cloves garlic, minced

- 2 cups baby spinach leaves

- 1 can (14 oz) diced tomatoes

- 1 teaspoon cumin

- 1 teaspoon paprika

- Salt and pepper to taste

- 2 cups vegetable broth

## Instructions:

1. In a pot, sauté onions and garlic until softened.

2. Add chickpeas, diced tomatoes, cumin, paprika, salt, and pepper.

3. Pour in vegetable broth and bring to a simmer.

4. Add baby spinach and cook until wilted.

5. Simmer for an additional 10 minutes before serving.

**Nutritional Information:**

- Chickpeas provide plant-based protein and fiber.
- Spinach is rich in vitamins and minerals.
- Tomatoes contribute antioxidants and flavor without acidity.

Recipe 12: Baked Cod with Lemon Herb Crust

**Ingredients:**

- 4 cod fillets
- 2 tablespoons olive oil
- 1 tablespoon fresh parsley, chopped
- 1 tablespoon fresh dill, chopped
- Zest of 1 lemon
- Salt and pepper to taste
- Lemon wedges for serving

**Instructions:**

1. Preheat the oven to 400°F (200°C).
2. Place cod fillets on a baking sheet.
3. In a bowl, mix olive oil, chopped parsley, chopped dill, lemon zest, salt, and pepper.
4. Spread the herb mixture over the cod fillets.
5. Bake for 15-20 minutes or until the fish is opaque and flakes easily.
6. Serve with lemon wedges.

## Nutritional Information:

- Cod is a lean protein source that is easy to digest.
- Olive oil provides heart-healthy fats.
- Fresh herbs and lemon add flavor without acidity.

## Recipe 13: Stuffed Bell Peppers with Quinoa and Black Beans

### Ingredients:

- 4 bell peppers, halved and seeds removed
- 1 cup cooked quinoa
- 1 can (15 oz) black beans, drained and rinsed
- 1 cup corn kernels (fresh or frozen)
- 1 cup diced tomatoes
- 1 teaspoon cumin
- 1 teaspoon chili powder
- Salt and pepper to taste
- 1/2 cup shredded plant-based cheese (optional)

### Instructions:

1. Preheat the oven to 375°F (190°C).
2. In a bowl, combine cooked quinoa, black beans, corn, diced tomatoes, cumin, chili powder, salt, and pepper.
3. Stuff each bell pepper half with the quinoa mixture.
4. If using, sprinkle shredded plant-based cheese on top.
5. Bake for 25-30 minutes or until the peppers are tender.

**Nutritional Information:**

- Quinoa and black beans provide plant-based protein and fiber.
- Bell peppers offer vitamins and are gentle on the stomach.
- Corn adds natural sweetness without acidity.

Recipe 14: Mango Ginger Chia Seed Pudding

**Ingredients:**

- 1/4 cup chia seeds
- 1 cup coconut milk
- 1 ripe mango, diced
- 1 teaspoon fresh ginger, grated
- 1 tablespoon maple syrup
- Toasted coconut flakes for topping

**Instructions:**

1. In a bowl, mix chia seeds and coconut milk. Let it sit for 10 minutes.
2. Stir in diced mango, grated ginger, and maple syrup.
3. Cover and refrigerate for at least 2 hours or overnight.
4. Before serving, stir the pudding and top with toasted coconut flakes.

**Nutritional Information:**

- Chia seeds provide omega-3 fatty acids and fiber.
- Coconut milk adds creaminess without dairy.
- Mango and ginger add flavor and digestive benefits.

## Ingredients:

- 4 boneless, skinless chicken breasts
- Zest and juice of 1 lemon
- 2 tablespoons fresh basil, chopped
- 2 tablespoons olive oil
- Salt and pepper to taste

## Instructions:

1. Preheat the grill or grill pan over medium-high heat.
2. In a bowl, mix lemon zest, lemon juice, chopped basil, olive oil, salt, and pepper.
3. Brush the mixture over both sides of each chicken breast.
4. Grill for 6-7 minutes per side or until the chicken is cooked through.
5. Let it rest for a few minutes before serving.

## Nutritional Information:

- Chicken is a lean protein source that is easy to digest.
- Lemon adds flavor without acidity.
- Basil contributes a fresh and aromatic element.



## Ingredients:

- 1 cup dried red lentils, rinsed
- 1 onion, chopped
- 2 carrots, diced
- 2 celery stalks, diced

- 3 cloves garlic, minced

- 1 teaspoon turmeric

- 1 teaspoon ground cumin

- 6 cups vegetable broth

- Juice of 1 lemon

- Fresh cilantro for garnish

**Instructions:**

1. In a pot, sauté onions, carrots, and celery until softened.

2. Add garlic, turmeric, and cumin. Stir for 1-2 minutes.

3. Add red lentils and vegetable broth.

4. Bring to a boil, then reduce heat and simmer for 20-25 minutes until lentils are tender.

5. Stir in lemon juice.

6. Garnish with fresh cilantro before serving.

**Nutritional Information:**

- Red lentils provide plant-based protein and fiber.

- Turmeric has anti-inflammatory properties.

- Lemon adds a burst of vitamin C without acidity.

## Recipe 17: Baked Herb-Crusted Turkey Breast

**Ingredients:**

- 1 boneless turkey breast

- 2 tablespoons olive oil

- 1 tablespoon fresh rosemary, chopped

- 1 tablespoon fresh thyme, chopped

- 1 teaspoon garlic powder

- Salt and pepper to taste

**Instructions:**

1. Preheat the oven to 375°F (190°C).

2. In a small bowl, mix olive oil, rosemary, thyme, garlic powder, salt, and pepper.

3. Rub the herb mixture over the turkey breast.

4. Place the turkey on a baking sheet and bake for 25-30 minutes or until cooked through.

5. Let it rest before slicing.

**Nutritional Information:**

- Turkey is a lean protein source that is easy to digest.

- Olive oil provides heart-healthy fats.

- Fresh herbs add flavor without triggering acidity.

## Recipe 18: Spinach and Mushroom Quiche with Oat Crust

**Ingredients:**

- 1 cup rolled oats

- 2 tablespoons olive oil

- 1 onion, diced

- 2 cups fresh spinach, chopped

- 1 cup mushrooms, sliced

- 4 large eggs

- 1 cup almond milk

- Salt and pepper to taste

## Instructions:

1.  Preheat the oven to 350°F (175°C).
2.  In a food processor, blend oats until they resemble flour.
3.  Mix oat flour with olive oil and press into a pie dish for the crust.
4.  In a skillet, sauté onions, spinach, and mushrooms until softened.
5.  Spread the vegetable mixture over the oat crust.
6.  In a bowl, whisk together eggs, almond milk, salt, and pepper. Pour over the vegetables.
7.  Bake for 30-35 minutes or until the quiche is set.

## Nutritional Information:

- Oats provide fiber for digestive health.
- Spinach and mushrooms offer vitamins and minerals.
- Almond milk is a dairy-free alternative that is gentle on the stomach.

## Recipe 19: Coconut Ginger Carrot Soup

## Ingredients:

- 4 cups carrots, chopped
- 1 onion, chopped
- 2 tablespoons fresh ginger, grated
- 1 can (14 oz) coconut milk
- 4 cups vegetable broth
- 2 tablespoons olive oil
- Salt and pepper to taste

## Instructions:

1. In a pot, sauté onions and ginger in olive oil until fragrant.
2. Add chopped carrots, coconut milk, and vegetable broth.
3. Bring to a boil, then reduce heat and simmer for 20-25 minutes until carrots are tender.
4. Use an immersion blender to blend the soup until smooth.
5. Season with salt and pepper to taste before serving.

## Nutritional Information:

- Carrots provide beta-carotene and are easy to digest.
- Ginger aids digestion and has anti-inflammatory properties.
- Coconut milk adds creaminess without dairy.

## Recipe 20: Buckwheat Banana Pancakes

## Ingredients:

- 1 cup buckwheat flour
- 1 teaspoon baking powder
- 1/2 teaspoon cinnamon
- 1 ripe banana, mashed
- 1 cup almond milk
- 1 tablespoon maple syrup
- Coconut oil for cooking

**Instructions:**

1.  In a bowl, mix buckwheat flour, baking powder, and cinnamon.

2.  In a separate bowl, combine mashed banana, almond milk, and maple syrup.

3.  Add the wet ingredients to the dry ingredients and stir until just combined.

4.  Heat coconut oil in a pan over medium heat.

5.  Spoon batter onto the pan to form pancakes and cook until bubbles form on the surface.

6.  Flip and cook until both sides are golden brown.

**Nutritional Information:**

- Buckwheat is a gluten-free whole grain that is gentle on the stomach.

- Banana adds natural sweetness and potassium.

- Almond milk is a dairy-free alternative.

These recipes are nutrient-rich as they incorporate a variety of colorful vegetables, whole grains, and plant-based protein sources. They are designed to support overall health, provide essential nutrients, and offer digestive comfort, making them suitable for individuals embracing plant-based nutrition and managing hiatal hernias.

# A ONE WEEK MEAL PLAN

Here's a one-week meal plan for the Hiatal Hernia Diet, focusing on gentle, nutrient-rich foods that support digestive health:

**Day 1:**

- **Breakfast:** Oatmeal with sliced bananas and a sprinkle of chia seeds.

- **Lunch:** Grilled chicken breast with steamed broccoli and quinoa.

- **Snack:** Greek yogurt with honey and a handful of almonds.

- **Dinner:** Baked salmon with lemon and dill, accompanied by roasted sweet potatoes.

**Day 2:**

- **Breakfast:** Buckwheat banana pancakes with a side of mixed berries.

- **Lunch:** Spinach and mushroom quiche with an oat crust.

- **Snack:** Carrot sticks with hummus.

- **Dinner:** Coconut ginger carrot soup with a side of whole-grain toast.

**Day 3:**

- **Breakfast:** Smoothie with fresh pineapple, kale, ginger, and coconut water.

- **Lunch:** Stuffed bell peppers with quinoa and black beans.

- **Snack:** Mango and avocado salad with lime dressing.

- **Dinner:** Baked herb-crusted turkey breast with a side of sautéed green beans.

**Day 4:**

- **Breakfast:** Chia seed pudding with almond milk and mixed berries.

- **Lunch:** Lentil and vegetable soup with a slice of whole-grain bread.

- **Snack:** Apple slices with almond butter.

- **Dinner:** Lemon basil grilled chicken with a quinoa and vegetable stir-fry.

**Day 5:**

- **Breakfast:** Greek yogurt parfait with granola and sliced strawberries.

- **Lunch:** Chickpea and spinach stew with a side of brown rice.

- **Snack:** Minty cucumber and melon salad.

- **Dinner:** Baked cod with a lemon herb crust, served with asparagus.

**Day 6:**

- **Breakfast:** Whole-grain toast with avocado and poached eggs.

- **Lunch:** Quinoa and vegetable stir-fry with tofu.

- **Snack:** Trail mix with nuts and dried fruits.

- **Dinner:** Turmeric lentil soup with a side of whole-grain crackers.

**Day 7:**

- **Breakfast:** Mango ginger chia seed pudding.

- **Lunch:** Grilled vegetable and hummus wrap in a whole-grain tortilla.

- **Snack:** Sliced cucumber with tzatziki.

- **Dinner:** Stuffed acorn squash with wild rice and cranberries.

**General Tips:**

- Stay hydrated throughout the day by drinking water or herbal teas.

- Consider smaller, more frequent meals to avoid overeating and minimize pressure on the stomach.

- Pay attention to portion sizes to prevent discomfort.

- Limit or avoid carbonated beverages, caffeine, and acidic foods that may trigger symptoms.

- Practice mindful eating, chewing food thoroughly, and eating in a relaxed environment.

Adjust the meal plan based on individual preferences, dietary needs, and any specific recommendations from a healthcare professional. It's essential to listen to your body and adjust as needed for optimal digestive comfort.

## The Delights of Organic and Gluten-Free Choices

Embracing a lifestyle centered around organic and gluten-free choices is not just a dietary preference; it's a commitment to nourishing your body with wholesome, unadulterated goodness. In the realm of food, these choices represent more than a trend – they encapsulate a philosophy that emphasizes health, sustainability, and a connection to the earth.

**Organic Bliss:**

Choosing organic foods is like inviting nature's best onto your plate. These offerings are cultivated without synthetic pesticides, herbicides, or genetically modified organisms (GMOs). It's a celebration of produce grown in nutrient-rich soil, under the gentle caress of the sun, and nurtured by the hands of mindful farmers. The result? Crisp, vibrant fruits and vegetables, and grains bursting with natural flavors, free from the residues of chemical interventions.

But it's not just about fruits and veggies – the organic lifestyle extends to the animal kingdom. Organic meats and dairy products come from animals raised in humane conditions, often with access to open pastures and a diet free from synthetic additives. Every bite becomes a nod to ethical farming practices and a pursuit of a healthier, more harmonious world.

**Gluten-Free Gastronomy:**

For those navigating the gluten-free journey, every meal becomes a dance of creativity. Gluten-free living is more than a dietary restriction; it's an exploration of alternative grains and a revelation of unexpected culinary gems. Imagine savoring a hearty bowl of quinoa or diving into the delicate intricacies of almond flour-based treats. These choices bring a newfound appreciation for the versatility and richness of gluten-free ingredients.

Moreover, for those with celiac disease or gluten sensitivity, a gluten-free lifestyle isn't just a preference – it's a necessity for well-being. It's about finding comfort in meals that don't trigger adverse reactions, paving the way for a life filled with vitality.

**The Symphony of Flavor:**

The beauty of organic and gluten-free choices lies not just in their health benefits but in the explosion of flavors they bring to your palate. Picture the succulence of an organically grown peach, its juices running down your chin, or the earthy aroma of gluten-free bread freshly baked, promising a satisfying crunch.

In this culinary symphony, the absence of artificial additives allows the true essence of each ingredient to shine. It's a celebration of purity, where the simplicity of a dish transforms into a gastronomic masterpiece.

**A Mindful Journey:**

Choosing organic and gluten-free options is a journey of mindfulness – a conscious decision to prioritize well-being and the well-being of the planet. It's about understanding the impact of our food choices on our bodies, the environment, and the community at large.

As you explore the delights of organic and gluten-free living, relish the fact that every bite is a step towards a healthier you and a healthier world. It's not just a diet; it's a lifestyle that harmonizes with the rhythms of nature and embraces the true essence of what it means to savor the delights of the earth.

## Recipes for Organic and Gluten-free choices:

Here are ten delicious recipes that embrace the delights of organic and gluten-free choices. Each recipe comes with instructions and nutritional information:

### Recipe 1: Quinoa-Stuffed Bell Peppers

**Ingredients:**

- 4 large bell peppers, halved and seeds removed
- 1 cup organic quinoa, cooked
- 1 can (15 oz) organic black beans, drained and rinsed
- 1 cup organic corn kernels
- 1 cup organic cherry tomatoes, diced
- 1/2 cup organic cilantro, chopped
- 1 teaspoon ground cumin
- 1 teaspoon smoked paprika
- Salt and pepper to taste
- 1 cup organic shredded cheese (optional)

**Instructions:**

1. Preheat the oven to 375°F (190°C).
2. In a bowl, mix cooked quinoa, black beans, corn, cherry tomatoes, cilantro, cumin, smoked paprika, salt, and pepper.
3. Stuff each bell pepper half with the quinoa mixture.
4. If using, sprinkle shredded cheese on top.
5. Bake for 25-30 minutes or until peppers are tender.
6. Serve with a dollop of organic Greek yogurt if desired.

**Nutritional Information:**

- Rich in protein and fiber from quinoa and black beans.

- Packed with vitamins and antioxidants from organic vegetables.

- Provides essential minerals like magnesium and iron.

Recipe 2: Organic Grilled Chicken Salad

**Ingredients:**

- 2 organic chicken breasts

- 6 cups organic mixed salad greens

- 1 cup organic cherry tomatoes, halved

- 1 organic cucumber, sliced

- 1/2 cup organic red onion, thinly sliced

- 1/4 cup organic feta cheese, crumbled

- Organic olive oil and balsamic vinegar for dressing

- Salt and pepper to taste

**Instructions:**

1. Season chicken breasts with salt and pepper and grill until fully cooked.

2. Slice the grilled chicken into strips.

3. In a large bowl, combine salad greens, cherry tomatoes, cucumber, red onion, and grilled chicken.

4. Drizzle with olive oil and balsamic vinegar.

5. Toss gently and sprinkle with crumbled feta.

6. Serve immediately.

## Nutritional Information:

- High-quality protein from organic chicken.
- Abundant vitamins and minerals from organic vegetables.
- Healthy fats from organic olive oil and feta cheese.

### Recipe 3: Gluten-Free Zucchini Noodles with Pesto

## Ingredients:

- 4 medium organic zucchinis, spiralized into noodles
- 1 cup organic cherry tomatoes, halved
- 1/2 cup organic pine nuts
- 2 cups organic basil leaves
- 1/2 cup organic Parmesan cheese, grated
- 2 cloves organic garlic
- 1/2 cup organic extra-virgin olive oil
- Salt and pepper to taste

## Instructions:

1. In a food processor, combine pine nuts, basil, Parmesan, and garlic. Pulse until finely chopped.
2. With the processor running, slowly pour in olive oil until a smooth pesto forms.
3. In a large pan, sauté zucchini noodles until just tender.
4. Toss zucchini noodles with cherry tomatoes and pesto.
5. Season with salt and pepper to taste.
6. Serve warm, garnished with extra pine nuts and Parmesan.

## Nutritional Information:

- Low-carb and gluten-free alternative to traditional pasta.

- Healthy fats from pine nuts and olive oil.

- Rich in vitamins and antioxidants from organic basil and tomatoes.

## Recipe 4: Organic Berry Smoothie Bowl

## Ingredients:

- 1 cup organic mixed berries (strawberries, blueberries, raspberries)

- 1 organic banana

- 1/2 cup organic Greek yogurt

- 1 tablespoon organic chia seeds

- 1 tablespoon organic honey

- Organic granola for topping

## Instructions:

1. Blend mixed berries, banana, Greek yogurt, chia seeds, and honey until smooth.

2. Pour the smoothie into a bowl.

3. Top with organic granola and additional berries.

4. Drizzle with a bit of honey for extra sweetness.

5. Enjoy with a spoon!

## Nutritional Information:

- Packed with antioxidants from organic berries.

- Probiotics from organic Greek yogurt for gut health.

- Omega-3 fatty acids from chia seeds.

# Recipe 5: Gluten-Free Almond Flour Banana Bread

**Ingredients:**

- 2 cups organic almond flour
- 1 teaspoon baking soda
- 1/2 teaspoon salt
- 3 ripe organic bananas
- 3 organic eggs
- 1/4 cup organic coconut oil, melted
- 1/4 cup organic honey
- 1 teaspoon organic vanilla extract

**Instructions:**

1. Preheat the oven to 350°F (175°C) and grease a loaf pan.
2. In a bowl, whisk together almond flour, baking soda, and salt.
3. In another bowl, mash the ripe bananas.
4. Add eggs, melted coconut oil, honey, and vanilla extract to the mashed bananas. Mix well.
5. Combine the wet and dry ingredients until a batter forms.
6. Pour the batter into the prepared loaf pan.
7. Bake for 50-60 minutes or until a toothpick comes out clean.
8. Allow the banana bread to cool before slicing.

**Nutritional Information:**

- Gluten-free alternative to traditional banana bread.

- Almond flour provides protein and healthy fats.

- Natural sweetness from ripe organic bananas.



**Ingredients:**

- 1 cup organic quinoa, cooked

- 1 cup organic cherry tomatoes, halved

- 1 cucumber, diced

- 1/2 cup organic Kalamata olives, sliced

- 1/4 cup organic red onion, finely chopped

- 1/2 cup organic feta cheese, crumbled

- Fresh parsley, chopped

- For the Lemon Vinaigrette:

    - 1/4 cup organic extra-virgin olive oil

    - Juice of 1 lemon

    - 1 teaspoon organic Dijon mustard

    - Salt and pepper to taste

**Instructions:**

1. In a large bowl, combine cooked quinoa, cherry tomatoes, cucumber, olives, red onion, and feta cheese.

2. In a separate small bowl, whisk together the ingredients for the lemon vinaigrette.

3. Drizzle the vinaigrette over the quinoa mixture and toss gently.

4. Garnish with fresh parsley.

5. Serve chilled.

**Nutritional Information:**

- Protein-packed quinoa.

- Vitamins and antioxidants from organic vegetables.

- Healthy fats from olive oil.

### Recipe 7: Gluten-Free Cauliflower Pizza Crust

**Ingredients:**

- 1 small organic cauliflower, riced

- 1 cup organic mozzarella cheese, shredded

- 1 organic egg

- 1 teaspoon organic dried oregano

- 1 teaspoon organic garlic powder

- Salt and pepper to taste

- Gluten-free pizza sauce and toppings of your choice

**Instructions:**

1. Preheat the oven to 400°F (200°C) and line a baking sheet with parchment paper.

2. In a bowl, mix riced cauliflower, mozzarella cheese, egg, oregano, garlic powder, salt, and pepper.

3. Spread the mixture onto the prepared baking sheet, shaping it into a pizza crust.

4. Bake for 20-25 minutes or until the edges are golden.

5. Remove from the oven and add pizza sauce and toppings.

6. Bake for an additional 10-15 minutes or until the cheese is melted and bubbly.

7. Slice and enjoy!

## Nutritional Information:

- Low-carb and gluten-free pizza crust.

- Cruciferous goodness from cauliflower.

- Protein from organic mozzarella cheese.

### Recipe 8: Organic Stir-Fried Tofu with Vegetables

## Ingredients:

- 1 block organic extra-firm tofu, pressed and cubed

- 2 tablespoons organic tamari or gluten-free soy sauce

- 1 tablespoon organic sesame oil

- 1 tablespoon organic coconut oil

- 1 cup organic broccoli florets

- 1 bell pepper, sliced

- 1 carrot, julienned

- 2 cloves organic garlic, minced

- Organic green onions, chopped (for garnish)

## Instructions:

1. In a bowl, marinate tofu cubes in tamari or soy sauce for 15 minutes.

2. Heat coconut oil in a wok or large pan over medium-high heat.

3. Add marinated tofu and stir-fry until golden.

4. Push tofu to one side and add sesame oil to the empty space.

5. Sauté garlic, then add broccoli, bell pepper, and carrot. Stir-fry until vegetables are tender-crisp.

6. Combine tofu and veggies, toss until well mixed.

7. Garnish with chopped green onions.

8. Serve over organic brown rice or quinoa.

## Nutritional Information:

- Plant-based protein from organic tofu.

- Nutrient-rich organic vegetables.

- Healthy fats from sesame and coconut oil.

### Recipe 9: Gluten-Free Almond Butter Banana Muffins

## Ingredients:

- 2 cups organic almond flour

- 1 teaspoon baking soda

- 1/4 teaspoon salt

- 3 ripe organic bananas, mashed

- 2 organic eggs

- 1/3 cup organic almond butter

- 1/4 cup organic honey

- 1 teaspoon organic vanilla extract

- Organic sliced almonds for topping

## Instructions:

1. Preheat the oven to 350°F (175°C) and line a muffin tin with paper liners.

2. In a bowl, whisk together almond flour, baking soda, and salt.

3. In another bowl, mix mashed bananas, eggs, almond butter, honey, and vanilla extract until well combined.

4. Combine the wet and dry ingredients until a batter forms.

5. Spoon the batter into the muffin tin, filling each cup about two-thirds full.

6. Top each muffin with sliced almonds.

7. Bake for 18-20 minutes or until a toothpick comes out clean.

8. Allow the muffins to cool before serving.

## Nutritional Information:

- Gluten-free almond flour for a moist texture.

- Protein and healthy fats from almond butter.

- Natural sweetness from ripe organic bananas.

## Recipe 10: Organic Berry Chia Seed Popsicles

## Ingredients:

- 1 cup mixed organic berries (strawberries, blueberries, raspberries)

- 2 tablespoons organic chia seeds

- 1 tablespoon organic honey or maple syrup

- 1 cup organic coconut water

## Instructions:

1. In a blender, combine mixed berries, chia seeds, honey or maple syrup, and coconut water. Blend until smooth.

2. Pour the mixture into popsicle molds.

3.  Freeze for 4-6 hours or until fully set.

4.  Run the molds under warm water to release the popsicles.

5.  Enjoy the refreshing and nutritious popsicles!

**Nutritional Information:**

- Antioxidants from organic berries.

- Omega-3 fatty acids and fiber from chia seeds.

- Hydration from organic coconut water.

These recipes not only cater to an organic and gluten-free lifestyle but also celebrate the rich flavors and nutritional benefits that these choices bring to your table. Adjust portions and ingredients according to personal preferences and dietary needs. Enjoy the wholesome goodness!

## DIETARY ALLERGIES

in the context of a "hiatal hernia diet for over 40" refer to specific food sensitivities or allergic reactions that individuals with hiatal hernias, especially those over the age of 40, may experience. While a hiatal hernia primarily involves the displacement of the stomach into the chest cavity through the diaphragm, it can be associated with symptoms such as acid reflux, heartburn, and indigestion.

In managing a hiatal hernia through diet, individuals may need to consider dietary allergies or sensitivities that could exacerbate their symptoms. Here are some aspects to consider:

1. **Acidic Foods:**

    - Individuals with hiatal hernias may be sensitive to acidic foods, as these can contribute to increased stomach acidity and worsen symptoms. Common acidic foods include citrus fruits, tomatoes, and certain vinegars.

2. **Spicy Foods:**

    - Spicy foods can be irritating to the esophagus and stomach, potentially triggering acid reflux. Individuals with dietary allergies or sensitivities to spicy foods may need to avoid them to minimize discomfort.

3. **Caffeine and Chocolate:**

    - Caffeine can relax the lower esophageal sphincter, contributing to acid reflux.

Chocolate, which contains both caffeine and other compounds, may also be problematic for some individuals. Those with dietary allergies or sensitivities to caffeine or chocolate may need to limit or avoid these items.

4. **Processed and Fried Foods:**

   - Highly processed and fried foods can be harder to digest, potentially leading to bloating and discomfort. Individuals with dietary allergies or sensitivities to certain food additives or fried foods may find relief by choosing whole, unprocessed options.

5. **Gluten and Dairy:**

   - Some individuals may have sensitivities or allergies to gluten or dairy, which can contribute to digestive issues. Considering gluten-free and dairy-free options may be beneficial for those with known sensitivities.

6. **Individualized Triggers:**

   - It's essential for individuals to identify their personal triggers. While certain foods are commonly associated with aggravating hiatal hernia symptoms, the impact can vary from person to person. Keeping a food diary and noting symptoms can help pinpoint specific dietary allergies or sensitivities.

7. **Balanced and Nutrient-Rich Diet:**

   - In contrast, focusing on a balanced and nutrient-rich diet can be beneficial for overall digestive health. Including lean proteins, fruits, vegetables, and whole grains while avoiding known triggers can contribute to a diet that supports individuals with hiatal hernias.

It's crucial for individuals managing hiatal hernias, especially those over 40, to work closely with healthcare professionals, including dietitians or gastroenterologists, to create a personalized dietary plan. This plan should take into account any dietary allergies or sensitivities while promoting overall digestive wellness and minimizing symptoms associated with hiatal hernias.

## Food Allergies

Food allergies are immune system reactions triggered by specific proteins in certain foods. When individuals with food allergies consume these particular foods, their immune system identifies the proteins as harmful invaders, leading to an overreaction that results in various symptoms. Food allergies can range from mild to severe, and in some cases, they can be life-threatening.

**Common Food Allergens:**

1. **Milk:** Allergic reactions to milk can range from mild to severe. Common symptoms include hives, stomach cramps, diarrhea, and, in severe cases, anaphylaxis.

2. **Eggs:** Egg allergies are more common in children. Symptoms can include skin reactions, digestive issues, and respiratory problems.

3. **Peanuts:** Peanut allergies can cause severe reactions, including anaphylaxis. Symptoms may include swelling, difficulty breathing, and a drop in blood pressure.

4. **Tree Nuts:** Allergies to tree nuts like almonds, walnuts, and cashews can also lead to severe reactions. Symptoms are similar to peanut allergies.

5. **Soy:** Soy allergies can cause digestive issues, skin reactions, and, in rare cases, anaphylaxis.

6. **Wheat:** Wheat allergies can cause a range of symptoms, including hives, digestive problems, and respiratory issues. It's distinct from gluten intolerance or celiac disease.

7. **Fish:** Allergic reactions to fish can be severe. Symptoms may include swelling, difficulty breathing, and gastrointestinal problems.

8. **Shellfish:** Shellfish allergies can cause severe reactions similar to those of fish allergies.



1. **Skin Reactions:** Hives, eczema, redness, or swelling.

2. **Gastrointestinal Issues:** Nausea, vomiting, abdominal pain, or diarrhea.

3. **Respiratory Symptoms:** Sneezing, coughing, wheezing, shortness of breath, or nasal congestion.

4. **Cardiovascular Symptoms:** Rapid heartbeat, drop in blood pressure, or, in severe cases, anaphylaxis.

5. **Other Symptoms:** Fatigue, dizziness, or lightheadedness.

Managing Food Allergies:

1. **Avoidance:** The primary way to manage food allergies is to avoid the specific food or foods that trigger the allergic reaction.

2. **Reading Labels:** Individuals with food allergies need to carefully read food labels to identify potential allergens.

3. **Emergency Action Plan:** Those with severe food allergies, especially those prone to anaphylaxis, should have an emergency action plan, including the use of epinephrine.

4. **Medical Supervision:** Regular check-ups with healthcare professionals, including allergists, help manage and monitor food allergies.

5. **Education:** Educating oneself and others (family, friends, coworkers) about food allergies is crucial for creating a safe environment.

6. **Support Groups:** Joining support groups or seeking counseling can provide emotional support and helpful tips for managing food allergies.

It's important for individuals with food allergies to work closely with healthcare professionals to develop a comprehensive management plan tailored to their specific needs. Dietary restrictions, lifestyle adjustments, and emergency preparedness are all crucial components of managing food allergies effectively.

In the context of a "hiatal hernia diet for over 40," food allergies may not be directly related to the structural issue of a hiatal hernia itself, but they can play a role in exacerbating symptoms or causing discomfort for individuals managing hiatal hernias. Hiatal hernias primarily involve the displacement of the stomach into the chest cavity through the diaphragm, leading to symptoms such as acid reflux, heartburn, and indigestion.

Here's how food allergies may connect to a hiatal hernia diet for individuals over the age of 40:

1. **Exacerbation of Acid Reflux:**

   - Certain foods that commonly trigger allergies, such as acidic or spicy foods, may also contribute to acid reflux symptoms associated with hiatal hernias. Individuals with food allergies to these types of foods may need to be especially cautious to avoid aggravating their symptoms.

2. **Digestive Discomfort:**

   - Individuals with hiatal hernias often experience digestive discomfort, and certain food allergies can exacerbate these issues. For example, those with lactose intolerance may find that dairy products contribute to bloating and gas, which can be uncomfortable for individuals with hiatal hernias.

3. **Individualized Triggers:**

   - Just as there is considerable variation in how different individuals respond to specific foods, the same holds true for those managing hiatal hernias. Some people may find that certain allergenic foods, even if not directly related to the hiatal hernia, can trigger or worsen symptoms such as heartburn or indigestion.

4. **Consideration of Dietary Restrictions:**

   - Individuals with known food allergies should take into account their dietary restrictions when planning a hiatal hernia-friendly diet. For example, if someone is allergic to gluten or dairy, they may need to choose alternative options that align with both their food allergies and the requirements of a hiatal hernia diet.

5. **Personalized Approach:**

   - Managing a hiatal hernia often involves a personalized approach to dietary choices. This includes considering individual tolerances and avoiding foods that may contribute to discomfort. If someone has food allergies, this becomes an additional layer of consideration in crafting a diet plan that supports overall digestive health.

It's essential for individuals over 40 with hiatal hernias to work closely with healthcare professionals, including dietitians, to create a personalized dietary plan. This plan should take into account any known food allergies, sensitivities, or triggers to ensure that the diet not only addresses hiatal hernia symptoms but also aligns with the individual's overall health and well-being.

# CHAPTER SIX

# CONVENIENCE MEETS HEALTH: SNACKS AND MEAL REPLACEMENTS

## Healthy Snack Options for Busy Lifestyles

Healthy snack options can play a crucial role in supporting individuals with a hiatal hernia, especially for those over the age of 40. Hiatal hernias can lead to symptoms such as acid reflux and indigestion, and making mindful choices when it comes to snacks can help alleviate discomfort and promote overall digestive health. Here's how healthy snack options can work for individuals with a hiatal hernia diet:

1. **Non-Acidic Fruits:**

   - Opt for non-acidic fruits such as bananas, melons, and pears as snacks. These fruits are less likely to trigger acid reflux and are gentle on the stomach.

2. **Low-Fat Dairy Alternatives:**

   - For individuals without lactose intolerance or dairy allergies, low-fat dairy alternatives like yogurt or kefir can be good snack choices. These options can provide probiotics, which may support digestive health.

3. **Whole Grains:**

   - Choose whole grains such as oatmeal, whole grain crackers, or rice cakes for snacks. Whole grains are generally well-tolerated and can provide a source of fiber without causing excessive stomach discomfort.

4. **Nuts and Seeds:**

- Opt for nuts and seeds, such as almonds or chia seeds, as snacks. They are rich in healthy fats and can provide a satisfying crunch without contributing to acid reflux.

5. **Vegetables with Hummus:**

   - Snack on non-acidic vegetables like carrot sticks, cucumber slices, or bell peppers with hummus. Hummus is a good source of plant-based protein and can be a flavorful addition without causing digestive issues.

6. **Smoothies:**

   - Prepare smoothies with non-acidic fruits, non-citrus berries, spinach, and a base of almond milk or other non-dairy alternatives. Smoothies can be a convenient and nutritious option, especially when avoiding acidic ingredients.

7. **Lean Protein:**

   - Snack on lean protein sources such as grilled chicken or turkey slices. Protein can help promote a feeling of fullness and may be less likely to trigger acid reflux compared to fatty or fried snacks.

8. **Herbal Teas:**

   - Choose non-acidic herbal teas like chamomile or ginger tea. These can be soothing for the digestive system and are a good alternative to acidic or caffeinated beverages.

9. **Avocado on Whole Grain Toast:**

   - Spread avocado on whole grain toast for a satisfying and nutritious snack. Avocado provides healthy fats, and whole grain toast offers fiber without being too heavy on the stomach.

10. **Hydration with Water:**

- Stay well-hydrated with water throughout the day. Adequate hydration is essential for overall digestive health and can help prevent dehydration, which may contribute to discomfort.

It's important for individuals with hiatal hernias to pay attention to their body's responses and identify specific triggers that may worsen symptoms. While the above snack options are generally well-tolerated, individual preferences and sensitivities vary. Consulting with a healthcare professional or a registered dietitian can provide personalized guidance based on an individual's specific health needs and dietary requirements.

# Meal Replacement Strategies for Sustainable Living

Meal replacement strategies for sustainable living can be adapted to support individuals with hiatal hernias, especially those over the age of 40. Hiatal hernias may cause symptoms such as acid reflux and indigestion, and making mindful choices when it comes to meal replacements can contribute to sustainable and comfortable eating habits. Here are some strategies to consider:

1. **Smoothies and Shakes:**

   - Prepare smoothies or shakes with non-acidic fruits, leafy greens, and a protein source such as plant-based protein powder or Greek yogurt. Smoothies can be nutrient-dense, easily digestible, and customizable based on individual preferences.

2. **Nutrient-Rich Soups:**

   - Choose nutrient-rich soups with a variety of vegetables, lean proteins, and whole grains. Soups provide hydration and can be well-tolerated by individuals with hiatal hernias. Opt for broth-based soups over creamy options to minimize fat content.

3. **Protein-Packed Salad Bowls:**

   - Create protein-packed salad bowls with lean proteins (chicken, turkey, tofu), non-acidic vegetables, and a variety of greens. Avoid acidic dressings and opt for olive oil or other non-acidic alternatives.

4. **Whole Grain Wraps or Sandwiches:**

- Use whole grain wraps or bread to create sandwiches with lean protein, non-acidic vegetables, and a spread like avocado. Be mindful of condiments, opting for those that are non-acidic and well-tolerated.

5. **Yogurt Parfaits:**

   - As a meal replacement or snack, prepare yogurt parfaits with non-acidic fruits, nuts, and seeds. Greek yogurt provides protein and can be easier on the stomach than dairy alternatives.

6. **Plant-Based Bowls:**

   - Build plant-based bowls with a base of quinoa or rice, a variety of cooked and raw non-acidic vegetables, and a plant-based protein source such as beans or lentils. Top with a non-acidic dressing.

7. **Oatmeal or Porridge:**

   - Choose oatmeal or porridge as a nutritious and filling meal replacement. Customize with non-acidic fruits, nuts, and seeds. Oats are a good source of soluble fiber, which can aid digestion.

8. **Egg-Based Meals:**

   - Incorporate egg-based meals such as omelets or scrambled eggs with non-acidic vegetables. Eggs provide protein and can be a versatile and easily digestible option.

9. **Non-Acidic Stir-Fries:**

  - Prepare stir-fries with non-acidic vegetables, lean proteins, and a base of rice or noodles. Use non-acidic sauces for flavoring.

10. **Homemade Energy Bars:**

  - Create homemade energy bars using ingredients like oats, nuts, seeds, and dried fruits. These can serve as convenient and portable meal replacements.

When adopting meal replacement strategies, it's important to consider individual tolerances and preferences. Pay attention to portion sizes and avoid overeating to minimize the risk of triggering hiatal hernia symptoms. Additionally, staying hydrated with water throughout the day is crucial for digestive health.

Individuals with hiatal hernias should consult with healthcare professionals, including dietitians, to create a sustainable meal plan tailored to their specific needs and dietary requirements. These strategies not only support digestive comfort but also contribute to overall well-being in the context of sustainable living.

# CHAPTER SEVEN
# SUPPORTIVE PRODUCTS FOR HIATAL HERNIA

## Hernia Belts and Truss Binders: An Overview

Hiatal hernias, particularly in individuals over the age of 40, can pose challenges that extend beyond dietary considerations. Managing the symptoms often requires a comprehensive approach. In addition to adopting a suitable hiatal hernia diet, individuals may explore supportive tools like hernia belts and truss binders to enhance their comfort and overall well-being.

**Understanding Hiatal Hernias:** Before delving into hernia belts and truss binders, it's crucial to understand hiatal hernias. These occur when part of the stomach protrudes into the chest through the diaphragm, leading to symptoms like acid reflux, heartburn, and indigestion. While dietary changes play a vital role, additional support may be sought through non-invasive devices like hernia belts.

## Hernia Belts:

Hernia belts, designed specifically for hiatal hernias, are supportive garments worn around the torso. They provide gentle compression, helping to keep the protruding stomach in place and alleviate symptoms. For individuals over 40 adhering to a hiatal hernia diet, these belts offer additional support during daily activities.

## Features and Benefits:

- **Adjustable Compression:** Most hernia belts are adjustable, allowing individuals to customize the level of compression based on their comfort and needs.

- **Comfortable Fabric:** Made from breathable materials, these belts are designed to be comfortable for extended wear, making them suitable for daily use.

- **Posture Support:** Some hernia belts provide added benefits by supporting proper posture, which can contribute to overall digestive comfort.

- **Activity Enhancement:** Individuals can wear these belts during various daily activities, offering support without hindering movement.

**Truss Binders:** Truss binders, like hernia belts, are supportive devices designed to hold the herniated tissue in place. While hernia belts are more versatile in terms of design, truss binders often have a more targeted approach, providing direct support to the affected area.

**Features and Benefits:**

- **Focused Support:** Truss binders typically have a targeted design, providing specific support to the herniated area, which can be beneficial for individuals with hiatal hernias.

- **Secure Fit:** Many truss binders come with adjustable straps or bands, ensuring a secure and personalized fit for the individual's comfort.

- **Minimized Discomfort:** By offering direct support to the herniated area, truss binders can help minimize discomfort during movement and various activities.

**Integration with hiatal hernia diet for over 40:**
- **Comfort during Meals:** Wearing a hernia belt or truss binder may provide added comfort during and after meals, aligning with the principles of a hiatal hernia diet.

- **Enhanced Mobility:** The supportive nature of these devices allows individuals to maintain their mobility, encouraging an active lifestyle, which is often recommended in conjunction with dietary changes.

- **Post-Meal Support:** After consuming a meal, individuals may experience increased pressure on the herniated area. Hernia belts and truss binders offer post-meal support, promoting comfort during digestion.

While dietary adjustments are pivotal in managing hiatal hernias, the integration of supportive devices like hernia belts and truss binders can complement these efforts. They provide an additional layer of support for individuals over 40, promoting comfort, mobility, and overall well-being as they navigate the challenges of hiatal hernia management alongside their chosen diet plan. Consulting with healthcare professionals is advisable to determine the most suitable approach for each individual's unique needs.

## Nature's Reveal: Vegetarian Capsules and Natural Dietary Supplements

In the pursuit of holistic well-being for individuals managing hiatal hernias, dietary supplements play a crucial role. Among them, vegetarian capsules and natural dietary supplements stand out for their compatibility with diverse diets, particularly those tailored for individuals over the age of 40 with hiatal hernias.

**Vegetarian Capsules:** Vegetarian capsules are an alternative to traditional gelatin capsules, offering a plant-based option that aligns with various dietary preferences, including vegetarian and vegan diets.

**Features and Benefits:**

1. **Plant-Based Composition:** Vegetarian capsules are typically made from cellulose, derived from plant sources like tapioca or pine.

2. **Digestive Compatibility:** For individuals with hiatal hernias, whose digestive systems may be sensitive, vegetarian capsules can be gentler on the stomach compared to some animal-based alternatives.

3. **Suitable for Dietary Preferences:** As more people adopt vegetarian or vegan lifestyles, the use of vegetarian capsules ensures that dietary supplements can accommodate diverse dietary choices.

4. **Reduced Allergen Risk:** Vegetarian capsules eliminate concerns related to common allergens present in gelatin, making them a suitable choice for those with allergies or sensitivities.

**Natural Dietary Supplements:** Natural dietary supplements complement the hiatal hernia diet for individuals over 40 by providing targeted nutrients that may be challenging to obtain solely from food sources.

Key Components:

1. **Digestive Enzymes:** Supplements containing digestive enzymes can aid in the breakdown of food, potentially reducing the burden on the digestive system and alleviating symptoms associated with hiatal hernias.

2. **Probiotics:** Supporting gut health is crucial for individuals with hiatal hernias. Probiotic supplements contribute beneficial bacteria to the digestive system, fostering a healthy gut microbiome.

3. **Anti-Inflammatory Ingredients:** Natural supplements may include anti-inflammatory compounds such as turmeric or ginger, which can help manage inflammation associated with hiatal hernias.

4. **Vitamins and Minerals:** Hiatal hernia management often involves addressing nutritional deficiencies. Supplements containing essential vitamins and minerals contribute to overall health and well-being.

## Integration into hiatal hernia diet for over 40:

1. **Comprehensive Support:** Vegetarian capsules containing natural dietary supplements offer a comprehensive approach to support individuals over 40 managing hiatal hernias, addressing both dietary and nutritional needs.

2. **Easy Incorporation:** Supplements in capsule form are convenient to incorporate into daily routines, ensuring consistent intake alongside dietary adjustments.

3. **Customizable Solutions:** With a variety of natural dietary supplements available, individuals can tailor their supplement regimen based on specific symptoms and nutritional requirements.

4. **Reduced Digestive Strain:** The gentle nature of vegetarian capsules and the use of natural ingredients in dietary supplements can contribute to reduced digestive strain, supporting individuals in their overall wellness journey.

Nature's reveal through vegetarian capsules and natural dietary supplements offers a harmonious integration with the hiatal hernia diet for individuals over 40. By combining the benefits of plant-based capsules and targeted nutritional support, individuals can enhance their holistic approach to managing hiatal hernias, promoting comfort, nutritional balance, and overall well-being. As with any dietary changes or supplement additions, consulting with healthcare professionals is advisable to ensure personalized and safe choices tailored to individual health needs.

# CHAPTER EIGHT
# DAILY ACTIVITIES AND FAST RECOVERY TIPS

## Holistic Recovery: Integrating Daily Activities

Holistic recovery for individuals managing hiatal hernias involves more than dietary changes; it extends to a comprehensive approach that incorporates various aspects of daily life. Integrating daily activities into a holistic recovery plan is crucial for promoting overall well-being and minimizing the impact of hiatal hernia symptoms. Here's an exploration of how holistic recovery can be achieved by seamlessly integrating daily activities:

1. **Mindful Eating Practices:**

   - **Explanation:** Adopting mindful eating practices involves being fully present during meals, savoring each bite, and paying attention to hunger and fullness cues.

   - **Integration:** Practice mindful chewing, enjoy the flavors of your hiatal hernia-friendly meals, and avoid distractions like electronic devices during meals.

2. **Posture Awareness:**

   - **Explanation:** Poor posture can contribute to hiatal hernia symptoms. Maintaining proper posture supports optimal digestion and reduces the risk of triggering discomfort.

   - **Integration:** Be mindful of your posture while sitting and standing. Sit up straight, avoid slouching, and consider activities like yoga or gentle stretches to improve overall posture.

3. **Regular Physical Activity:**

- **Explanation:** Exercise is essential for overall health, including digestive health. Regular physical activity promotes circulation, reduces stress, and supports a healthy weight.

- **Integration:** Choose low-impact exercises such as walking, swimming, or yoga that align with your fitness level. Aim for consistency rather than intensity, and consult with healthcare professionals for personalized exercise recommendations.

4. **Stress Management Techniques:**

   - **Explanation:** Stress can exacerbate hiatal hernia symptoms. Implementing stress management techniques helps reduce the impact of stress on the digestive system.

   - **Integration:** Explore stress-reducing activities such as deep breathing exercises, meditation, or hobbies that bring joy and relaxation. Establish a daily routine that includes moments of mindfulness.

5. **Adequate Hydration:**

   - **Explanation:** Proper hydration supports overall digestive health and helps prevent dehydration, which can contribute to discomfort.

   - **Integration:** Drink water throughout the day, especially between meals. Limit the consumption of carbonated and caffeinated beverages, as they may contribute to acid reflux.

6. **Quality Sleep:**

   - **Explanation:** Sleep is crucial for the body's healing and recovery processes. Poor sleep can impact digestion and exacerbate hiatal hernia symptoms.

   - **Integration:** Establish a consistent sleep routine, create a comfortable sleep environment, and prioritize getting enough rest each night.

7. **Listening to Body Signals:**

   - **Explanation:** Understanding and responding to the body's signals is fundamental in holistic recovery. Recognizing when to rest or when to engage in activities promotes balance.

   - **Integration:** Pay attention to signals of fatigue, discomfort, or stress. Adjust your daily activities accordingly, allowing for periods of rest and relaxation.

8. **Social Connections:**

   - **Explanation:** Emotional well-being is interconnected with physical health. Maintaining social connections and engaging in positive interactions contribute to overall holistic recovery.

   - **Integration:** Foster social relationships, whether through virtual or in-person interactions. Share your journey with supportive friends or family members.

Holistic recovery, when applied to managing hiatal hernias, entails a harmonious integration of daily activities that nurture physical, mental, and emotional well-being. By adopting mindful practices, maintaining a healthy lifestyle, and prioritizing self-care, individuals can optimize their recovery journey and enhance their overall quality of life. Consulting with healthcare professionals can provide personalized guidance on integrating daily activities into a holistic recovery plan tailored to individual health needs.

# Tips For Fast Recovery and Overall Well-Being in Hiatal Hernia Management

Recovering from a hiatal hernia involves a holistic approach that encompasses dietary changes, lifestyle modifications, and mindful practices. These tips aim to promote fast recovery and overall well-being for individuals managing hiatal hernias:

1. **Adherence to a Hiatal Hernia Diet:**

   - **Explanation:** Follow a hiatal hernia-friendly diet that emphasizes non-acidic and easily digestible foods. This includes lean proteins, whole grains, fruits, and vegetables.

   - **Integration:** Plan well-balanced meals, avoid trigger foods, and eat smaller, more frequent meals to reduce pressure on the stomach.

2. **Mindful Eating Practices:**

   - **Explanation:** Adopt mindful eating habits to enhance digestion and prevent overeating. Chew food slowly, savor each bite, and be attuned to hunger and fullness cues.

   - **Integration:** Create a calm eating environment, minimize distractions, and focus on the sensory experience of eating.

3. **Hydration Habits:**

   - **Explanation:** Stay adequately hydrated with water between meals. Proper hydration supports digestion and helps prevent dehydration-related discomfort.

   - **Integration:** Carry a water bottle, set hydration goals, and limit the intake of caffeinated and carbonated beverages that can contribute to acid reflux.

4. **Gentle Exercise Routine:**

   - **Explanation:** Engage in low-impact exercises that promote overall health without exacerbating hiatal hernia symptoms. Activities like walking, swimming, or yoga are beneficial.

   - **Integration:** Develop a consistent exercise routine, incorporating activities that align with your fitness level. Consult with healthcare professionals for personalized exercise recommendations.

5. **Posture Awareness:**

   - **Explanation:** Maintain proper posture to alleviate pressure on the stomach and reduce the risk of triggering hiatal hernia symptoms.

   - **Integration:** Sit and stand up straight, avoid slouching, and consider posture-improving exercises or practices like yoga.

6. **Stress Management Techniques:**

   - **Explanation:** Stress can worsen hiatal hernia symptoms. Implement stress management techniques to reduce its impact on the digestive system.

   - **Integration:** Practice deep breathing exercises, meditation, or engage in activities that promote relaxation and emotional well-being.

7. **Adequate Sleep Routine:**

- **Explanation:** Quality sleep is essential for the body's healing processes. Poor sleep can impact digestion and overall recovery.

- **Integration:** Establish a consistent sleep schedule, create a comfortable sleep environment, and prioritize sufficient hours of rest each night.

8. **Regular Medical Check-ups:**

- **Explanation:** Schedule regular check-ups with healthcare professionals, including gastroenterologists and dietitians, to monitor progress and make necessary adjustments to the treatment plan.

- **Integration:** Communicate openly with healthcare providers, share any changes in symptoms, and follow their guidance for ongoing management.

9. **Social Support:**

- **Explanation:** Emotional well-being is integral to overall health. Maintain social connections and share your journey with supportive friends or family members.

- **Integration:** Seek support from loved ones, join support groups, and engage in positive social interactions to enhance emotional resilience.

10. **Individualized Approach:**

- **Explanation:** Every individual's journey with hiatal hernia is unique. Pay attention to your body's signals, adjust your lifestyle based on personal needs, and customize your recovery plan.

- **Integration:** Reflect on how specific lifestyle choices impact your symptoms and make informed adjustments. Collaborate with healthcare professionals to tailor your approach to individual health needs.

By integrating these tips into daily life, individuals managing hiatal hernias can promote fast recovery and overall well-being. It's essential to approach recovery holistically, considering both physical and emotional aspects, and to work closely with healthcare professionals to ensure a personalized and effective recovery plan.

## Addressing Unique Needs for Women in Hiatal Hernia Management

Hiatal hernias can present unique challenges for women, especially as they age. Recognizing and addressing these distinctive needs is crucial for effective management and overall well-being. Here are key considerations tailored to address the unique needs of women in hiatal hernia management:

1. **Hormonal Influences:**

   - **Explanation:** Hormonal fluctuations, particularly during menstruation, pregnancy, and menopause, can impact digestive health and exacerbate hiatal hernia symptoms.

   - **Addressing Needs:** Women should be mindful of their hormonal cycles and work with healthcare professionals to adapt dietary and lifestyle strategies accordingly during different life stages.

2. **Pregnancy and Hiatal Hernia:**

   - **Explanation:** Pregnancy can exert additional pressure on the abdomen, potentially worsening hiatal hernia symptoms. Hormonal changes during pregnancy may also contribute to acid reflux.

   - **Addressing Needs:** Pregnant women with hiatal hernias should work closely with healthcare providers to manage symptoms, adjust their diet, and explore safe and effective interventions.

3. **Menopausal Changes:**

   - **Explanation:** Menopausal hormonal shifts may impact digestion and increase the risk of gastrointestinal symptoms. Women may experience changes in weight distribution and metabolism.

   - **Addressing Needs:** Menopausal women should focus on maintaining a healthy weight, adopting lifestyle measures to manage symptoms, and consulting with healthcare professionals for personalized guidance.

4. **Bone Health Considerations:**

   - **Explanation:** Women are more prone to osteoporosis, and certain medications prescribed for hiatal hernias, such as proton pump inhibitors, may impact bone health.

   - **Addressing Needs:** Women should prioritize bone health through adequate calcium and vitamin D intake, weight-bearing exercises, and regular bone density assessments.

5. **Nutritional Requirements:**

   - **Explanation:** Women may have specific nutritional needs, especially related to iron, calcium, and vitamin B12, which can be influenced by dietary restrictions or medications used for hiatal hernia management.

   - **Addressing Needs:** Women should work with dietitians to ensure their hiatal hernia-friendly diet meets nutritional requirements, considering age-related changes and potential deficiencies.

6. **Pelvic Floor Health:**

   - **Explanation:** Pelvic floor health can be influenced by hiatal hernias, and women may experience pelvic floor dysfunction alongside hernia symptoms.

   - **Addressing Needs:** Pelvic floor exercises, under the guidance of healthcare professionals, can contribute to better pelvic floor health, potentially alleviating symptoms and improving overall well-being.

7. **Post-Surgical Considerations:**

   - **Explanation:** Women may undergo hiatal hernia surgery, and post-surgical care can be influenced by factors such as reproductive health, recovery during menstruation, and considerations for future pregnancies.

   - **Addressing Needs:** Women should communicate their reproductive health goals with their surgical team to tailor post-surgical care and ensure optimal recovery.

8. **Psychosocial Support:**

   - **Explanation:** Women often play multiple roles, and the psychosocial impact of hiatal hernias can affect their daily lives, relationships, and mental health.

   - **Addressing Needs:** Women should seek psychosocial support, engage in open communication with healthcare providers about the emotional aspects of their journey, and consider counseling or support groups.

9. **Breast Health Screening:**

- **Explanation:** Women, particularly those in midlife and beyond, should prioritize regular breast health screenings. Some medications for hiatal hernias may require consideration in screening protocols.

- **Addressing Needs:** Coordinate with healthcare providers to ensure that hiatal hernia medications do not interfere with breast health screenings, and maintain regular mammograms and breast self-exams.

10. **Individualized Care Plans:**

- **Explanation:** Women's health is diverse, and individualized care plans should consider factors such as reproductive health, family planning, and unique lifestyle needs.

- **Addressing Needs:** Women should actively participate in the development of personalized care plans, collaborating with healthcare professionals to address their specific concerns and goals.

By acknowledging and addressing these unique needs, women can navigate hiatal hernia management more effectively, promoting better symptom control, improved quality of life, and enhanced overall well-being. Regular communication with healthcare professionals and a proactive approach to health maintenance are essential components of this tailored strategy.

# Customized Support for Female Hiatal Hernia Patients

Supporting female patients with hiatal hernias requires a personalized and nuanced approach that considers their unique needs and experiences. Here's a guide on how to provide customized support for female hiatal hernia patients:

1. **Holistic Assessment:**

    - **Explanation:** Begin by conducting a thorough assessment that takes into account not only the physical symptoms but also the patient's hormonal, reproductive, and psychosocial factors.

    - **Implementation:** Work closely with the patient to understand her overall health, lifestyle, and any specific concerns related to her female anatomy.

2. **Tailored Dietary Guidance:**

    - **Explanation:** Recognize the impact of hormonal fluctuations on digestive health. Tailor dietary recommendations to address hormonal changes during menstruation, pregnancy, and menopause.

    - **Implementation:** Collaborate with a registered dietitian to create a hiatal hernia-friendly diet plan that aligns with the patient's hormonal cycles and nutritional needs.

3. **Pregnancy-Related Considerations:**

    - **Explanation:** Acknowledge the influence of pregnancy on hiatal hernia symptoms. Provide guidance on managing symptoms during pregnancy and explore safe interventions.

- **Implementation:** Work closely with obstetricians to ensure coordinated care, adjusting medications or dietary recommendations as needed during pregnancy.

4. **Menopausal Support:**

- **Explanation:** Address the digestive changes that may accompany menopause. Consider the potential impact of hormonal therapy on hiatal hernia symptoms.

- **Implementation:** Collaborate with gynecologists to integrate digestive health considerations into menopausal management, ensuring a holistic approach to overall well-being.

5. **Nutritional Counseling:**

- **Explanation:** Recognize potential nutrient deficiencies in women, such as iron or calcium, and tailor nutritional counseling to meet these specific needs.

- **Implementation:** Conduct regular nutritional assessments and collaborate with a dietitian to design a nutrient-rich diet that supports overall health and addresses potential deficiencies.

6. **Pelvic Floor Health Integration:**

   - **Explanation:** Understand the interplay between hiatal hernias and pelvic floor health, which may be particularly relevant for women.

   - **Implementation:** Collaborate with pelvic health specialists to incorporate pelvic floor exercises or physical therapy into the patient's treatment plan for comprehensive care.

7. **Psychosocial Support:**

   - **Explanation:** Recognize the psychosocial impact of hiatal hernias on women, considering the potential stressors related to multiple roles and societal expectations.

   - **Implementation:** Encourage open communication, and consider referrals to mental health professionals or support groups to address the emotional aspects of living with a chronic condition.

8. **Breast Health Coordination:**

   - **Explanation:** Acknowledge the importance of breast health for women. Ensure that medications prescribed for hiatal hernias do not interfere with breast health screenings.

   - **Implementation:** Coordinate with breast health professionals to align screening schedules, and educate the patient on the importance of regular breast health examinations.

9.  **Reproductive Health Dialogue:**

- **Explanation:** Initiate discussions about reproductive health goals, family planning, and the potential impact of hiatal hernia management on fertility or pregnancy.

- **Implementation:** Engage in open conversations, involve reproductive health specialists as needed, and tailor care plans to align with the patient's family planning preferences.

10. **Individualized Care Plans:**

- **Explanation:** Recognize that every woman's experience with hiatal hernias is unique. Develop individualized care plans that consider specific concerns, preferences, and lifestyle factors.

- **Implementation:** Involve the patient in decision-making, set realistic goals, and adjust care plans as needed to accommodate changes in health or life circumstances.

Customized support for female hiatal hernia patients involves a collaborative and empathetic approach. By acknowledging the diverse needs of women and tailoring care plans accordingly, healthcare providers can enhance the patient's experience, improve symptom management, and contribute to their overall well-being.

## Understanding the Importance of Optimum Elasticity

In the realm of hiatal hernia management, recognizing the significance of optimum elasticity becomes paramount, particularly when considering supportive devices, lifestyle modifications, and overall well-being. Here's an exploration of why optimum elasticity is crucial in the context of hiatal hernias:

1. **Supportive Garments:**

   - **Explanation:** Optimum elasticity in supportive garments, such as hernia belts and truss binders, ensures a snug yet flexible fit. This elasticity provides gentle compression, helping to keep the stomach in place without causing discomfort.

   - **Importance:** Proper support aids in symptom management, prevents exacerbation of hernia-related issues, and promotes overall comfort during daily activities.

2. **Breathability and Comfort:**

   - **Explanation:** Fabrics with optimal elasticity allow for breathability and comfort. This is particularly important for individuals with hiatal hernias, as excess pressure or constriction can lead to increased discomfort.

   - **Importance:** Breathable and comfortable materials enhance the wearability of supportive garments, encouraging individuals to incorporate them into their daily routines for sustained relief.

3. **Mobility and Flexibility:**

   - **Explanation:** Optimum elasticity in garments and support devices facilitates natural body movement and flexibility. Restriction in mobility can be counterproductive, hindering regular activities and affecting overall well-being.

   - **Importance:** Unrestricted movement enables individuals to engage in daily tasks, exercise, and maintain an active lifestyle, contributing to both physical and mental health.

4. **Post-Meal Support:**

   - **Explanation:** After meals, the stomach may experience increased pressure, especially for individuals with hiatal hernias. Optimum elasticity in supportive devices allows for gentle compression during these periods without causing undue strain.

   - **Importance:** Post-meal support aids in digestion, minimizes the risk of hernia protrusion, and contributes to a more comfortable experience during and after eating.

5. **Customized Fit:**

   - **Explanation:** Adjustable elasticity in supportive devices allows for a customized fit tailored to individual body shapes and sizes. This adaptability ensures that the compression is distributed evenly, maximizing effectiveness.

- **Importance:** A customized fit enhances the efficacy of the supportive garment, providing targeted support to the herniated area while accommodating the unique contours of the wearer's body.

6. **Preventing Irritation:**

   - **Explanation:** Fabrics with optimum elasticity are less likely to cause irritation or chafing, which is crucial for individuals with hiatal hernias who may already experience sensitivity in the abdominal region.

   - **Importance:** Comfortable, irritation-free wear encourages consistent use of supportive garments, promoting adherence to the recommended care plan and contributing to long-term symptom management.

7. **Enhanced Compliance:**

   - **Explanation:** Supportive devices with optimal elasticity are more likely to be worn consistently. Compliance with wearing these devices is essential for achieving sustained benefits and managing hiatal hernia symptoms effectively.

   - **Importance:** When individuals find the supportive garments comfortable and accommodating, they are more likely to integrate them into their daily routines, leading to better overall compliance with the recommended care plan.

8. **Durability and Longevity:**

- **Explanation:** Fabrics with optimum elasticity tend to be more durable and resistant to wear and tear. This durability ensures that supportive garments maintain their effectiveness over an extended period.

- **Importance:** Long-lasting supportive devices provide ongoing relief, reducing the need for frequent replacements and contributing to a cost-effective and sustainable approach to hiatal hernia management.

Understanding the importance of optimum elasticity underscores its role in enhancing the effectiveness, comfort, and durability of supportive garments for hiatal hernia management. Whether in the context of post-meal support, personalized fit, or overall well-being, the right balance of elasticity contributes to a positive and supportive experience for individuals navigating the challenges of hiatal hernias.

# Lightweight Moisture-Wicking Fabric for Comfort

In the realm of hiatal hernia management, the choice of materials in supportive garments, particularly those made from lightweight moisture-wicking fabric, holds a pivotal role in enhancing comfort and overall well-being. This discussion explores the significance of this fabric choice and its positive impact on individuals navigating the challenges of hiatal hernias.

1. **Understanding Hiatal Hernia Challenges:**

   - **Context:** Hiatal hernias, involving the protrusion of the stomach through the diaphragm, can cause discomfort, reflux, and digestive issues. Managing these challenges requires a multifaceted approach, including supportive garments to alleviate symptoms and enhance daily comfort.

2. **The Role of Supportive Garments:**

   - **Context:** Supportive garments, such as hernia belts and truss binders, play a crucial role in providing gentle compression, reducing strain on the herniated area, and supporting overall abdominal stability.

   - **Significance:** Choosing the right fabric for these garments becomes paramount, and lightweight moisture-wicking fabric emerges as a key consideration for optimal comfort.

3. **Lightweight Construction:**

   - **Context:** Lightweight fabrics are designed to be thin and breathable, minimizing the feeling of bulkiness or constriction. This is particularly important for individuals with hiatal hernias who may already experience sensitivity in the abdominal region.

- **Significance:** The lightweight nature of the fabric ensures that individuals can wear supportive garments discreetly under clothing without sacrificing comfort or mobility.

4. **Moisture-Wicking Properties:**

- **Context:** Moisture-wicking fabrics are engineered to draw moisture away from the body, promoting evaporation and keeping the skin dry. This is especially beneficial for individuals who may experience perspiration or discomfort in the abdominal area.

- **Significance:** By efficiently managing moisture, these fabrics contribute to a drier and more comfortable environment, reducing the risk of skin irritation and enhancing overall wearability.

5. **Enhanced Breathability:**

- **Context:** Breathability is a critical factor in the comfort of supportive garments. Fabrics with good breathability allow air circulation, preventing overheating and maintaining a comfortable temperature.

- **Significance:** Lightweight moisture-wicking fabric promotes enhanced breathability, ensuring that individuals can wear supportive garments for extended periods without feeling excessively hot or uncomfortable.

6. **Reducing Friction and Irritation:**

- **Context:** Friction and irritation can be concerns, especially in the abdominal region where supportive garments come into direct contact with the skin. Lightweight moisture-wicking fabrics are designed to minimize friction.

- **Significance:** By reducing friction and irritation, these fabrics contribute to a smoother and more comfortable wearing experience, encouraging consistent use of supportive garments.

7. **Flexibility and Freedom of Movement:**

- **Context:** The flexibility of the fabric is crucial for maintaining freedom of movement. Individuals with hiatal hernias should be able to go about their daily activities without feeling restricted by their supportive garments.

- **Significance:** Lightweight moisture-wicking fabrics provide the necessary flexibility, allowing individuals to move comfortably and engage in regular activities without compromising the effectiveness of the supportive garment.

8. **Promoting Daily Adherence:**

- **Context:** Adherence to wearing supportive garments is essential for managing hiatal hernia symptoms effectively. Comfort plays a pivotal role in encouraging individuals to wear these garments consistently.

- **Significance:** Lightweight moisture-wicking fabric contributes to a positive wearing experience, promoting daily adherence and ensuring that individuals can experience the ongoing benefits of the supportive garment.

9. **Choosing Sustainable Materials:**

   - **Context:** The choice of fabric also extends to sustainability considerations. Opting for lightweight moisture-wicking fabrics that are durable and easy to care for aligns with a sustainable approach to hiatal hernia management.

   - **Significance:** Sustainable materials contribute to the longevity of supportive garments, reducing the environmental impact and providing individuals with a reliable and eco-friendly solution for their ongoing needs.

   Lightweight moisture-wicking fabric emerges as a pivotal choice in elevating the comfort of supportive garments for individuals managing hiatal hernias.

   **Closing Thoughts:** By prioritizing materials that are lightweight, moisture-wicking, and conducive to breathability, individuals can experience not only effective symptom management but also a level of comfort that enhances their overall quality of life. The right fabric choice becomes an integral part of a holistic approach to hiatal hernia management, ensuring that individuals can navigate their daily lives with confidence and ease.

# CONCLUSION
# EMBRACE YOUR WELLNESS JOURNEY

## Recap of Key Dietary and Lifestyle Strategies

Hiatal hernia management involves a holistic approach that integrates dietary and lifestyle strategies to alleviate symptoms and enhance overall well-being. Here's a recap of key strategies:

1. **Hiatal Hernia-Friendly Diet:**

   - *Explanation:* Adopt a diet that focuses on non-acidic and easily digestible foods.

   - *Importance:* Minimizes reflux and discomfort associated with hiatal hernias.

2. **Mindful Eating Practices:**

   - *Explanation:* Embrace mindful chewing, savoring each bite, and paying attention to hunger and fullness cues.

   - *Importance:* Supports digestion and prevents overeating, reducing pressure on the stomach.

3. **Hydration Habits:**

   - *Explanation:* Stay adequately hydrated with water between meals.

   - *Importance:* Supports digestion, prevents dehydration-related discomfort, and aids overall well-being.

4. **Gentle Exercise Routine:**

   - *Explanation:* Engage in low-impact exercises like walking, swimming, or yoga.

- *Importance:* Promotes overall health without exacerbating hiatal hernia symptoms.

5. **Posture Awareness:**

   - *Explanation:* Maintain proper posture to alleviate pressure on the stomach.

   - *Importance:* Reduces the risk of triggering hiatal hernia symptoms.

6. **Stress Management Techniques:**

   - *Explanation:* Practice stress-reducing activities such as deep breathing exercises and meditation.

   - *Importance:* Mitigates the impact of stress on the digestive system.

7. **Adequate Sleep Routine:**

   - *Explanation:* Establish a consistent sleep schedule and prioritize sufficient hours of rest.

   - *Importance:* Supports the body's healing processes and overall recovery.

8. **Regular Medical Check-ups:**

   - *Explanation:* Schedule regular check-ups with healthcare professionals.

   - *Importance:* Monitors progress, allows for adjustments to the treatment plan, and ensures overall health.

9. **Social Support:**

   - *Explanation:* Foster social connections and engage in positive interactions.

- *Importance:* Enhances emotional well-being and provides a support system.

10. **Individualized Care Plans:**

- *Explanation:* Tailor care plans to individual needs, considering factors like hormonal influences and reproductive health.

- *Importance:* Addresses unique challenges and preferences, optimizing overall management.

11. **Lightweight Moisture-Wicking Fabric:**

- *Explanation:* Choose supportive garments made from lightweight, moisture-wicking fabric.

- *Importance:* Enhances comfort, breathability, and wearability of supportive devices.

12. **Optimum Elasticity:**

- *Explanation:* Prioritize supportive garments with optimum elasticity for a customized and comfortable fit.

- *Importance:* Provides gentle compression, supports abdominal stability, and ensures flexibility in movement.

13. **Breathability and Comfort:**

- *Explanation:* Opt for materials that allow breathability and minimize friction.

- *Importance:* Reduces discomfort, encourages consistent use of supportive garments, and promotes overall well-being.

14. **Customized Support for Women:**

- *Explanation:* Acknowledge and address unique needs related to hormonal influences, pregnancy, menopause, and pelvic floor health in women.

- *Importance:* Tailors care plans to individual experiences, promoting effective management and overall comfort.

15. **Understanding the Basics of Hiatal Hernia Diet:**

- *Explanation:* Gain a clear understanding of why dietary choices matter.

- *Importance:* Provides foundational knowledge for individuals seeking long-term benefits from dietary changes.

16. **Long-term Benefits of Making Dietary Changes:**

- *Explanation:* Explore the extended advantages of incorporating dietary changes into one's life.

- *Importance:* Reinforces the commitment to a hiatal hernia-friendly lifestyle for sustained well-being.

These strategies collectively form a comprehensive approach to hiatal hernia management. By integrating these principles into daily life, individuals can navigate the challenges of hiatal hernias with greater ease, promoting symptom relief and improving their overall quality of life.

# Peyton Audrey's Encouragement for A Holistic Approach to Hiatal Hernia Management

Dear Friends,

Embarking on a journey to manage hiatal hernia brings both challenges and opportunities for positive change. As your guide and advocate on this path, I encourage you to embrace a holistic approach that not only addresses the physical aspects of this condition but also nurtures your mind, body, and soul.

## 1. Acknowledging Your Unique Journey:

- *Embrace Your Uniqueness:* Your journey with hiatal hernia is unlike anyone else's. Embrace your uniqueness and recognize that your body requires an individualized approach to healing.

## 2. Peyton's Holistic Healing Strategies:

- *Mind-Body Connection:* Understand the intricate connection between your mind and body. Explore holistic healing strategies that encompass not just physical care but also mental and emotional well-being.

## 3. Incorporating Mind, Body, and Soul into Your Wellness Journey:

- *Mindfulness Practices:* Integrate mindfulness into your daily routine. Whether through meditation, deep breathing, or simply being present in the moment, mindfulness can alleviate stress and positively impact your overall well-being.

## 4. Comprehensive Table of Contents: Hiatal Hernia Diet for Over 40:

- *Knowledge is Power:* Dive into the comprehensive knowledge outlined in the book. Equip yourself with insights on dietary choices, lifestyle modifications, and the intricacies of hiatal hernia management.

## 5. Balanced Living:

- *Finding Balance:* Strive for balance in your life. This includes a balance between work and relaxation, physical activity and rest, and the foods that nourish your body.

## 6. Peyton Audrey's Recipes for Healing:

- *Nourishing Recipes:* Explore the recipes provided with the intention of nourishing your body. These recipes are not just about sustenance; they are a celebration of flavors that contribute to your overall well-being.

## 7. Peyton's Guidance on Individualized Care:

- *Tailored Care Plans:* Recognize the power of individualized care. Your journey is unique, and your care plan should reflect that uniqueness. Collaborate with healthcare professionals to tailor your approach.

## 8. Peyton's Insights on Long-Term Benefits:

- *Commit to Long-Term Wellness:* Understand the long-term benefits of the choices you make today. Commit to a lifestyle that promotes sustained well-being, not just short-term relief.

## 9. Encouragement for Daily Adherence:

- *Daily Commitment:* I encourage you to commit to your daily wellness routine. Adherence to supportive practices, dietary choices, and mindfulness will contribute to your overall success.

**10. Peyton's Holistic Healing Community:** - *Community Support:* Connect with others on a similar journey. Share your experiences, learn from one another, and foster a supportive community where everyone is empowered to thrive.

Remember, healing is a journey, not a destination. It's about progress, not perfection. Approach your hiatal hernia management with patience, self-compassion, and a belief in your body's innate ability to heal.

Wishing you holistic wellness and a journey filled with self-discovery and empowerment.

Warm regards, Peyton Audrey